Flat Belly Diet!

A BREAKTHROUGH PLAN

Flat Belly Diet !

LIZ VACCARIELLO AND CYNTHIA SASS

LOSE UP TO 15LB IN JUST 32 DAYS!

How to get the flat stomach you've always wanted.
(NOT A SINGLE SIT-UP REQUIRED.)

RODALE

First published 2009 by Rodale, an imprint of Pan Macmillan

This edition published 2010 by Rodale
an imprint of Pan Macmillan, a division of Macmillan Publishers Limited
Pan Macmillan, 20 New Wharf Road, London N1 9RR
Basingstoke and Oxford
Associated companies throughout the world
www.panmacmillan.com

ISBN 978-1-9057-4454-1

1 3 5 7 9 8 6 4 2

A CIP catalogue record for this book is available from the British Library.

Printed in the UK by CPI Mackays, Chatham ME5 8TD

Notice
This book is intended as a reference volume only, not as a medical manual. The information
given here is designed to help you make informed decisions about your health. It is not
intended as a substitute for any treatment that you may have been prescribed by your doctor.
If you suspect that you have a medical problem, we urge you to seek competent medical help.

The information in this book is meant to supplement, not replace, proper exercise training. All
forms of exercise carry some inherent risks. The editors and publisher advise readers to take full
responsibility of their safety and know their limits. Before practising the exercises in this book,
be sure that your equipment is well maintained, and do not take risks beyond your level of
experience, aptitude, training and fitness. The exercise programme in this book is not intended
as a substitute for any exercise routine that may have been prescribed by your doctor. As with all
exercise programmes, you should get your doctor's approval before beginning.

Mention of specific companies, organizations or authorities in this book does not imply
endorsement by the publisher, nor does mention of specific companies, organizations or
authorities in the book imply that they endorse the book, its author or the publisher.
Websites and telephone numbers given in this book were correct at the time of going to press.

Visit **www.panmacmillan.com** to read more about all our books and to buy them. You will
also find features, author interviews and news of any author events, and you can sign up for
e-newsletters so that you're always first to hear about our new releases.

LIVE YOUR WHOLE LIFE™

We inspire and enable people to improve their lives and the world around them

FOR THE MILLIONS WHO BEMOAN

THEIR BELLIES, SO THEY CAN

LEARN TO LOVE THEM INSTEAD.

Liz and Cynthia

contents

acknowle

dgments

We dedicate the *Flat Belly Diet* to the readers of *Prevention* – all 11 million of you – who have told us in no uncertain terms that belly fat is your biggest physical challenge.

Our gratitude to the Rodale family. For generations, through their magazines, books, and online properties, they have been committed to a special mission, that of giving people the tools and inspiration to live their whole lives. Our most heartfelt thanks to Rodale CEO Steve Murphy, whose leadership means Rodale is the kind of company where creativity is nurtured and the highest standards are set – and met – daily. It all starts with the edit, Steve!

Like magazines, books are a collaborative effort, and this one is no exception. Very special thanks to Gregg Michaelson ('Let's make it happen!'), Janine Slaughter, Liz Perl Erichsen and Jim Berra (the unsung hero behind all things *Prevention*). To Robin Shallow, who never met an idea she didn't improve, and Karen Mazzotta, who is tireless in her enthusiasm, support and belief in this plan. And to Fotoulla Euripidou, for her understanding of the *Prevention* audience and for helping us determine whether *Prevention* readers would be interested in this kind of diet book – by asking them!

We'd also like to extend our gratitude to the original members of our initial test panel, which was conducted in the summer of 2007. They first opened our eyes to how special the *Flat Belly Diet* really was. Thank you Mary Aquilar, Syndi Becker, Katherine Brechner, Donna Christiano, Evelyn Gomer, Diane Kastareck, Patti Lloyd, Kevin Martin, Nichole Michl, Colleen O'Neill-Groves, Julie Plavsic and Mary Anne Speshok for devoting your summer to this project and providing us with the essential insights that helped us develop this book beyond daily meal plans. Thank you also Gina Allchin, President, Health Trek P.T.T., who measured each and every one of our panellists with precision and compassion – a tough combination!

You would not be holding this book in your hands without executive editor Nancy Hancock ('good to great!'). All thanks to her dedicated team, including Chris Krogermeier, Marina Padakis, Anthony Serge, JoAnn Brader, Keith Biery, Hope Clarke, Wendy Gable and Ana Palmiero. And of course, to Ina Yalof – one of the fastest, most creative writers we've ever known – we offer a round of applause.

Big hugs to *Prevention*'s brilliant creative director, Jill Armus, whose ability to communicate elegance, authority and strength through colour and design have infused the entire *Prevention* brand of products (most recently this book cover and interior) with new vitality. And to *Prevention* fitness director Michele Stanten, whose contribution to and extensive review of Chapter 9 have helped make it one of the most authoritative sources of information on banishing belly fat with exercise.

Thanks also to Miriam Backes, Merritt Watts, Amy Gorin, Katie Kackenmeister and Kristen Watson, who assisted with co-ordinating the test panel and editing and fact-checking the manuscript, even during precious nights and weekends. To Lori Conte, Courtenay Smith and Polly Chevalier: for keeping the trains running on time. And to the smartest photo and art team in the business, including *Prevention*'s Helen Cannavale, Kim Latza, Faith Enemark, Jessica Sokol and Donna Agaja-nian. And of course to Rosalie Rung, who helped capture the enormous success of our test panellists on film and video.

Our deepest gratitude we save for brand editor Leah McLaughlin, a longtime colleague and friend to both of us. From helping develop the initial idea to making sure the most engaging, authoritative manuscript shipped to the printer and every moment in between, Leah was critical to the launch of this book.

Finally, we'd like to thank our husbands, Steve Vaccariello and Jack Bremen, and families (especially Olivia and Sophia Vaccariello and Diane Salvagno!) for putting up with all the late – late! – nights and never-ending conversations about *Flat Belly Diet* this and *Flat Belly Diet* that. (Yes, now we can take a weekend off, guys!)

1

GET READY FOR A FLAT BELLY

IT DOESN'T MATTER what your personal stumbling blocks are: baby weight, killer cravings or (say it with me) 'getting older'. Belly fat is *not* your destiny. I am delighted to tell you that you can, and will, get rid of it. The editors of *Prevention* magazine have found a way to target belly fat that is healthy, real, long-lasting and works for everyone.

Before we get started, I think it's important to do a 'gut check'. Chances are, if you've forked out your hard-earned cash for a book called *Flat Belly Diet*, you may wish you had someone else's belly or wish you had your own belly – from 20 years ago.

If that's you, I would ask you to change your thinking. Be kind to your belly. No matter how flat or round, jiggly or rock hard – it's yours, and it's powerful. It's probably the centre of some of your most profound memories. Think about it . . . the laughter you've shared, the romantic dinners you've had, the butterflies you've felt, the children you may have carried. All these set up house in – yes – your belly. And for that it deserves your respect. Your appreciation. And more than a little love and kindness . . . even when you're struggling to button up your jeans.

HOW DO I FEEL ABOUT MY BELLY? I consider it my core strength, and I love to feel it move, twist and support me as I go through life's business. It's where food (one of life's greatest pleasures, of course) touches down, and there are few things as peaceful for me as that not-stuffed-not-hungry-but-just-full feeling. It's also my meditative centre, and I sense the calm overtaking me when I fill my middle with deep breaths. Then, of course, there's the role it played in my pregnancy with twins. Anything willing to expand to host two precious, growing, kicking girls earns a special place in my heart for all time.

But the belly betrays. If I'm bloated the morning after a sushi dinner, that's where my outfit feels tight. If PMS strikes, my belly moans and groans. When I put on 5 pounds, that's where it shows. And, of course, when I try to take those 5 pounds off, that's where they stay.

As editor-in-chief of top US health magazine *Prevention*, one of the best things about my job is hearing from readers and learning – clearly and quickly – that I am not alone in my love/hate affair with this fascinating, troublesome part of the body. Many of you have told me that when you look at yourself in the mirror, you overlook your familiar, beautiful features, the favourite nuances of your physique. Instead, your eye travels directly to the areas where your fat resides. And, for most of us, that's the belly.

For countless reasons that I will outline throughout this book, the belly starts letting us down at around the age of 40. Some time between our 35th and 55th birthdays (some earlier, some later and some lucky ones never), the belly pouches, puffs and starts spilling over our waistbands. First we suck it in, yet it refuses to achieve its formerly flat shape. Then we crunch until our necks scream, while the fat over the sculpted abs muscles remains. And eventually we diet, then watch with frustration as the weight disappears from our breasts and our faces and the belly fat stays put. Eventually, belly fat starts to feel like our destiny – something that even hours on the treadmill or the strictest diet in the world won't budge. . .

Until now.

MY QUEST TO FIND THE BEST WAY to get rid of belly fat started when I took on *Prevention*'s nutrition director, Cynthia Sass. Her first challenge was to comb the latest research, combine it with her vast clinical experience and develop a diet that would target abdominal fat specifically. I made a good decision – Cynthia is not only a phenomenal magazine editor but also a registered dietitian with three university degrees and 15 years of experience, including countless hours of working with women in the real world. And here's the best part: she is passionate about food! I knew that any diet I asked her to construct would be satisfying and delicious, that it would be a way of eating that women could embrace for a lifetime. And wow, was I right.

She has developed a belly-shrinking eating plan that is grounded in the latest and most credible science (that you won't find anywhere else!) – and offers the most filling, satisfying and delicious meals that you will ever have the pleasure of eating.

But my vision for this *Flat Belly Diet* went beyond food. I know that any successful diet acknowledges that we eat for emotional reasons as well as physical ones. Not only does the *Flat Belly Diet* deliver a healthy, satisfying way of eating – one that will rid your body of fat in the place you told us you want to slim down most – but it will teach you how to *want* to eat this way for ever. The mental tricks, tips and strategies are culled from the latest research and are designed to inspire you, motivate you and set you up for a better relationship with food for the rest of your life!

Belly Fat Defined

WHEN I MENTION the words 'belly fat', I'm actually talking about two different types: *subcutaneous* and *visceral*, which collects centrally around your abdomen. **Subcutaneous fat** is best, though perhaps not most scientifically, defined as the fat that you can see, the 'inch you can pinch'. *Subcutaneous* means 'beneath' (*sub*) 'the skin' (*cutaneous*), and it's no big secret that this fat resides all over the body. In some spots – your thighs, underarms, *tummy, anyone?* – it may be thicker than in others, but for the most part it's everywhere, even on the soles of your feet. A moderate amount of subcutaneous fat is essential for life – for one thing, it keeps you from freezing to death in the winter. But too much of it causes dissatisfaction with how we look (which studies show leads to even more dangerous health behaviours). And worse: excessive amounts of subcutaneous fat function as a visible sign of being overweight or obese, which doctors know raises your risk for many diseases. But I have some great news: subcutaneous fat responds immediately to this diet plan.

Before you happily skip pages and move to the diet, let's talk about the second type of fat – visceral – which is much more dangerous and difficult to lose. **Visceral fat** resides deep within your torso and is sometimes referred to as 'hidden' belly fat. I prefer the term 'deadly'. Because of its proximity to your heart and liver, excess visceral fat can increase your risk of all sorts of diseases, from heart disease and diabetes to cancer and Alzheimer's. And the most frustrating part? You can cut calories and exercise religiously and still be left with too much of it.

In fact, the only way to minimize both visceral and subcutaneous fat simultaneously is to eat the right . . . fat.

The New Belly-Flattening Nutrient

WE'VE KNOWN ABOUT the benefits of monounsaturated fat – the kind found in olive oil, nuts and avocados – for decades. Nearly every health magazine contains some tip or strategy for getting more in your diet. In fact, we're on such intimate terms with monounsaturated fatty acids that we have a nickname for them – MUFAs (pronounced MOO-fahs). But it wasn't until the spring of 2007 that we realized just how amazing these fats are. That was when Spanish researchers published a study in the journal *Diabetes Care* showing that eating a diet rich in MUFAs *can actually help prevent weight gain in your belly.*[1]

The researchers looked at the effects of three different diets – one high in saturated fat, another high in carbohydrates and a third rich in MUFAs – on a group of patients with 'abdominal fat distribution', or, in language the rest of us non-scientists can understand, belly fat. All three diets contained the same number of calories, but only the MUFA diet was found to reduce the accumulation of belly fat and, more specifically, visceral belly fat.

Bear in mind: *no other nutrient can do this.* And that's what makes the *Flat Belly Diet* unlike any other diet book you've ever read. It presents the only diet to give MUFAs centre stage, to make them an essential part of every single meal. And that means it's the only diet that helps you lose fat in the belly *specifically*! In Chapter 3, you'll read more about MUFAs and their various health benefits, but until then, let's take a broader look at this truly groundbreaking diet plan.

The Flat Belly Diet Programme

THE FLAT BELLY DIET is made up of two parts – the *Four-Day Anti-Bloat Jumpstart* and the *Four-Week Eating Plan*. The whole thing together takes just 32 days, which studies show is just enough time to make any dietary change a lifestyle. Then, after you've mastered the programme and seen the desired changes in your weight and measurements, I give you the tools to keep your belly flat for life. Even though you may be tempted to follow one part without the other, I want you to start with the Anti-Bloat Jumpstart, then move straight into the Four-Week Eating Plan. Here's why.

■ THE FOUR-DAY ANTI-BLOAT JUMPSTART isn't just about beating bloat; it's also extremely important in sparking your emotional commitment to the whole programme. The 4-day plan includes a prescribed list of foods and drinks that will help flush out fluid, reduce water retention, and relieve digestive issues like wind and constipation, which can make your belly swell unnecessarily. You'll drink Cynthia's signature Sassy Water and eat healthy foods like fruits, vegetables and whole grains. When we tested this diet on our group of volunteers, one of the participants lost an amazing *7lb and 5 inches in the first 4 days (that's just 96 hours).*

Losing the bloat isn't just a way to fit into your favourite dress again. It's about feeling confident, powerful and proud of your body. Dropping even a few pounds of unnecessary water weight can be thrilling and can give you a major confidence boost – essential for success on any diet plan. Plus, I've added a second element to the 4-day plan: a Mind Trick at every meal. These quick and easy healthy-eating triggers will serve as mealtime reminders that you have embarked on a new way of life – a new way of living with and caring for your body.

What about Exercise?

I exercise every day, walking 50 minutes as part of my commute. (I also strength-train every weekend and try to fit in a weekly Pilates class or yoga session, too.) And I encourage everyone to make exercise a part of his or her lifestyle.

To that end, I asked *Prevention*'s fitness director Michele Stanten to devise the exercise programme in Chapter 9 for you to follow as you embark on the *Flat Belly Diet*. Adding a fitness programme to the eating plan and mental strategies will mean faster results (it certainly did for some of our testers).

But what makes the *Flat Belly Diet* truly special is that *you don't need to exercise to reap the benefits*. If you do exercise, you will certainly see results

■ THE FOUR-WEEK EATING PLAN begins the morning after you complete the Anti-Bloat Jumpstart, and it's the centrepiece of this book. Every day you'll enjoy three super satisfying 400-calorie meals and one 400-calorie Snack Pack. Each meal and snack contains just the right amount of MUFA to make that belly fat disappear. How simple is that? No calorie counting. No maths! We chose the quantity of 1,600 calories per day because that's the precise amount an adult woman of average height, frame, size and activity level needs to get down to her ideal body weight while maintaining a high energy level, healthy immune system and strong muscles. It also ensures you won't feel tired, irritable, moody or hungry.

But because no plan fits all, we've provided two different versions: the first one's perfect for people who have little time to spend in the kitchen. In Chapter 7, you'll find 70 different 400-calorie, MUFA-packed Quick-and-Easy-Fix Meals and 28 different 400-calorie Snack Pack options. Choose three meals and one Snack Pack a day and you're done. In a month, you'll have a flatter belly and I'll have done my job.

Sometimes, however, you'll want a more involved home-cooked meal, whether it's family night, or the weekend, or you're just a good cook who

faster, and you will gain secondary benefits like improved cardiovascular health and stronger, more toned muscles. But you can still expect to shrink your belly – and lose both subcutaneous and visceral fat – by simply following the eating plan.

If you do not already exercise regularly, you don't have to start doing so right away. I have always been a big believer in the phrase 'small changes, big results'. To me, it's more important that you do *something* to reduce your belly fat than it is to do *everything*, only to find that too many changes are too overwhelming to maintain. If you do not already have a workout routine, incorporating a new way of eating into your lifestyle may be change enough for the first 32 days.

likes to flex her culinary muscles now and then. In Chapter 8, you'll find more than 80 recipes that all provide the requisite number of calories and MUFAs per serving, so they can be swapped for any of your required three meals a day.

Throughout the programme, it's important to stay motivated. To help you, it's a good idea to start writing a journal for the 28 days. Track your own progress in this journal by recording your eating in a food diary, noting down weekly weight and measurements, as well as your mood changes to help control emotional eating. Recognizing the emotional connection with food is critical to losing weight and keeping it off. In your journal you can explore your relationship to food, and start to notice the reasons behind the way that you eat. Remember to read back over previous entries, as that way you can spot behaviour patterns and notice your progress. Writing down your reasons for sticking to the programme; for example, wanting to be able to wear a bikini for a beach holiday, or feeling energized enough to run around with your children, will remind you why you are doing it and ensure you feel inspired to succeed.

Throughout this book, look for the boxes entitled **Did You Know?** to learn more about fat, weight loss and general health. These are quick tips, strategies and bits of information that experts and readers tell me are useful. And don't forget to read the entries titled **Sass from Sass**. Cynthia wrote these to share her thoughts and advice about how to achieve success on this amazing programme. You'll also find incredible success stories from the women (and men) who participated in our *Flat Belly Diet* test panel – and who have a flatter belly to prove it!

If I know one thing for certain after years editing *Prevention* magazine, it's that maintaining a healthy mind and body are the most important things I can do for myself – and my family. I hope that by the time you finish reading this book and following this plan, you will have fallen in love with your flatter belly, your healthier, more wholesome way of eating and the amazing energy and vitality that come with better health!

Flat Belly Diet!

> The Four-Day Anti-Bloat Jumpstart

A full 96 hours is all it takes to spark your commitment to the *Flat Belly Diet* – and lose a few pounds! The Jumpstart consists of:

A DAILY DOSE OF SASSY WATER Created by Cynthia, this make-in-advance concoction helps guard against dehydration.

A MIND TRICK AT EVERY MEAL Fast mental fixes help get your brain in the Flat Belly game.

> The Four-Week Plan

Twenty-eight days of delicious MUFA-packed meals and recipes that you can mix and match. The plan consists of:

FOUR 400-CALORIE MEALS A DAY Choose from our meal selections or recipes, and be sure to make one meal a Snack Pack.

A MUFA AT EVERY MEAL These super-healthy fats keep you feeling full and ensure every meal is exceptionally tasty.

> An Optional Exercise Programme

Fat-burning walks, a Metabolism Boost and a Belly Routine will help you build muscle and maximize calorie burn.

My Flat Belly Success Story

Before:

Starting weight: _____

Starting waist measurement: _____

Starting hip measurement: _____

After:

Current weight: _____

Current waist measurement: _____

Current hip measurement: _____

READ A FLAT BELLY
SUCCESS
STORY

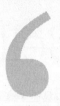

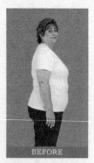

BEFORE

Mary Anne Speshok

AGE: 55

POUNDS LOST:

15
IN 32 DAYS

ALL-OVER
INCHES LOST:

10

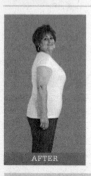

AFTER

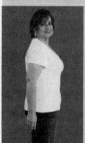

At press time:

3½
STONE
LOST
IN 5
MONTHS!

'I'M NOT A KID ANY MORE,' says 55-year-old Mary Anne Speshok. But you'd never know it from listening to her describe the effect of her new weight loss on her husband of 5 years. 'He's chasing me around the room! Like I'm his toy! He looks at me and says, "Wow! I can't believe what I'm seeing!"'

Mary Anne says her husband was as happy as she is with her results from the first 4 weeks on the *Flat Belly Diet*. In just 32 days, she had lost 3½ inches off her hips, 3½ off her stomach, 3 inches off her back (that little place that hangs over the bra strap) and an inch from each thigh. 'On the scales today, I lost 2 more pounds. I feel as if the weight is melting off of me. People tell me I'm walking with more confidence in my step. It's terrific!'

The administrative assistant has a message for anyone considering the *Flat Belly Diet*: 'The only thing you have to do is start it. All the tools are there.'

She calls it a revolutionary, do-able winner – do-able, she says, because the MUFAs keep you satisfied. 'Most people, including me, don't stick to a diet plan because they get hungry between meals. The difference with this diet is you literally don't get hunger pains. It's revolutionary because you start seeing results so fast that you want to keep going.' And the winner part? 'Well,' she adds, 'just look at what I've lost.'

Mary Anne has committed herself to doing the *Flat Belly* Workout in Chapter 9 along with the diet. Even though she works full-time and commutes an hour each way to and from work, she still manages to get in her paces. She usually walks for 30 minutes at lunchtime, but on days when she can't, she stops at the gym even before she goes home and does her 30 minutes of walking there. At home, she either does floor exercises or uses hand weights. She says her energy level is so high these days that exercising is easy.

And like so many recently thin women, Mary Anne has just discovered how great it is to fit into a nice, slim pair of jeans. 'I never even owned a pair before,' she says. 'I liked them, but just not on me.' Not any more, though. She says she just went out and bought three different styles of jeans because they all looked so good on her.

In fact, Mary Anne's wardrobe is getting a full workout these days. She's buying new clothes to fit her new body. And she's adding bracelets and necklaces, 'which I love. When I felt so big, I just wore my wedding ring and my watch. You don't want to call attention to yourself because you don't feel pretty. But now, bring on the jewellery! The more the better!' She and her husband are renewing their vows soon, and she's looking forward to wearing a beautiful gown that she hasn't been able to fit into for a long time. 'What a prize for reaching your goal,' she exclaims. 'To fit into something that hung in your wardrobe, just waiting. This beautiful gown . . . and a size smaller.'

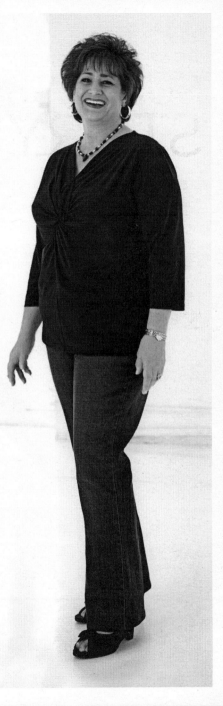

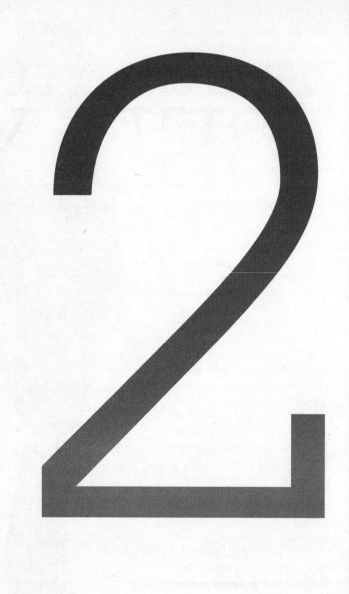

THE SKINNY ON
BELLY
FAT

BODY FAT IS ESSENTIAL. **Without it, you couldn't survive.** Your cells wouldn't be able to hold together or absorb nutrients from the food you ate. Your organs wouldn't be able to produce the hormones that make you distinctly female. You would freeze to death on a cold day. You'd run the risk of damaging your internal organs just by bumping into a doorknob. And forget ever finding your keys again. Without fat, your brain probably wouldn't even be able to work out what a key is.

In effect, *you* wouldn't be *you* without fat. Body fat, whether it's found on your thighs or buttocks or within the intricate coils of your brain, plays a role in nearly every single biological function in your body, and it's impossible to live without it. Of course, there's a fine line between having just the right amount of body fat and having too much.

The Trouble with Belly Fat

SCIENTISTS HAVE KNOWN for some time now that excess body fat isn't good for you. Obesity – which, technically speaking, means to be 'overfat' – is considered to be as deadly as smoking, according to some analyses. When you step on the scales, you're getting a rough indication of how heavy you are, but you can't tell how fat you are. The body mass index (BMI) gets you closer to working it out. Here's how to calculate it.

- Multiply your weight in pounds by 703.
- Divide that number by your height in inches.
- Divide that number by your height in inches again.

A woman who weighs 145 pounds (11stone 5lb) and is 67 inches tall (5ft 7in) has a BMI of 22.7. A woman who weighs 260 pounds (18stone 5lb) and is 67 inches tall has a BMI of 40.7.

If your BMI is 25 or higher, you're considered 'overweight', but if your BMI is 30 or above, you're 'obese'. If it's 40 or above, you're 'morbidly obese', and your health is at great risk. A BMI below 18.5 is 'underweight' – that's also cause for concern, because it indicates too low a percentage of body fat to ensure healthy functioning. An index between 18.5 and 24.9 is just right.

However, one of the problems with the body mass index is that it doesn't account for your muscle mass. As a result, some athletes – who have a much lower percentage of body fat and higher percentage of muscle – can compute to be overweight or, in some rare cases, obese.

More recently, studies have begun to show that while being obese in general is unhealthy, carrying excess body fat specifically *around your belly* is really, really unhealthy. Studies show that women who have waistlines measuring 35 inches or more are at greater risk for heart disease and diabetes than those whose waistline measurements are smaller. For men, a waistline measurement of 40 or above can be an indicator of the same health risks. Heart disease is the number one killer of women in England and Wales, and rates of diabetes have reached worrying levels. The connection between the measurement of your waist and your risk of dying from one of these diseases is no mere coincidence.

According to a study reported in the *New England Journal of Medicine*, people with large hips and small waists produce higher levels of HDL cholesterol, the protective form, than do those with large bellies.[1] (I like to remember the two types of cholesterol in this way: HDL is the 'healthy' kind, LDL is the 'lousy' kind.) Women typically have higher HDL levels – which is linked to fewer heart attacks – than men do. But that all changes after menopause, when body fat distribution changes due to hormone shifts and a woman's risk for heart attack increases.

If you're overweight or obese, take your pick of things to blame – creamy sauces, for one. Not to mention ice cream and soft drinks, and cakes and cheese and – well, you get the picture. Eating too much of any food can make you fat. Cutting back on cardiovascular exercise is another way to add inches all over, as is skipping a weight-training routine. And, for some of us, genetics plays a role. But something happens to us after the age of 40 that makes it easier to put on *belly fat* in particular: our hormones go haywire.

DID YOU KNOW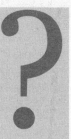

We're all born with the same number of fat cells (about 40 billion, give or take). As we grow up, the number of fat cells we have increases until after our pubescent and adolescent years, when they are pretty much set. In the past, it was assumed that the only difference between overweight people and thin ones was that overweight or obese people had all their fat cells filled to maximum capacity. It's now known that we can – and do, in fact – 'grow' more fat cells in adulthood. This is because when fat cells expand to their maximum size, they divide and increase again the number of fat cells. Some obese people have more fat cells than non-obese people. **But in the end, both the number and the size of the fat cells determine the amount of fat someone has.**

As oestrogen levels decline, your body struggles to maintain its hormonal balance. In the process, body fat – which is extremely important in manufacturing oestrogen and other sex hormones, not to mention preserving bone mass – becomes more valuable and thus harder to get rid of. As you approach the menopause, your body fat distribution starts to look more like a man's and less like a woman's.

What do I mean by that? Well, you've heard of the term *beer belly*? Male body fat tends to concentrate around the belly area – and it doesn't really have much to do with beer, except for the fact that, because beer is a source of excess calories, it's generally a catalyst for weight gain. Female body fat, on the other hand, tends to concentrate around the hips, thighs and buttocks during the years that we're most likely to reproduce. Some researchers theorize that as oestrogen levels decline, a woman's body stops laying down fat in these trouble zones and starts laying down fat near the belly, like a man's body does.

An LDL/HDL Primer

The UK National Institute for Health and Clinical Excellence (NICE) and Department of Health guidelines are that total cholesterol should be less than 5.0mmol/L (millimols per litre of blood) and LDL cholesterol should be less than 3.0mmol/L. There are several types of cholesterol, but in most cases, health professionals concentrate on two – namely, HDL and LDL. LDL is known as the 'bad' cholesterol because it builds up on artery walls and can lead to increased risk for cardiovascular disease and stroke. A level of 130 mg/dL (milligrams per deciliter of blood) or less is considered optimal for most people. HDL is the healthy cholesterol.

It transports LDL cholesterol out of the bloodstream and deposits it in the liver, where it can be processed and excreted. High amounts of HDL (60 mg/dL or higher) give some protection from heart disease.

The ratio of HDL to total cholesterol is a very good way of measuring cardiovascular risk. Most doctors consider a ratio of 4 or under excellent. A person with total cholesterol of 200 mg/dL and an HDL of 50 mg/dL (total/HDL ratio = 4) has a lower risk of heart disease and stroke than someone with a total of 180 mg/dL and an HDL of 30 mg/dL (total/HDL ratio = 6).

Not every woman ends up with excess midriff weight in middle age. Although some women with small waists and large hips can with time develop a midriff large enough that it becomes the broadest part of her body, other women keep the 'pear' shape for ever. For them, the weight gained in the midriff around the menopause is new, but subcutaneous fat is still stored in the hips, thighs or elsewhere.

V Is for Vicious

VISCERAL FAT GETS its name from the term *viscera*, which refers to the internal organs in the abdomen. It lies cloaked deep inside your body, where it wraps around your heart, liver and other nearby major organs. Because it's sequestered beneath a layer of muscle, and it doesn't jiggle when you walk or always show up in your girth, some people call it 'hidden fat'. In fact, it's possible to be relatively thin and still have too much visceral fat. But this kind of fat can do far more than add inches to your waist: it can subtract years from your life. Carrying excess visceral fat is one of a complex group of symptoms collectively called metabolic syndrome, or syndrome X. The other symptoms are high cholesterol, high blood pressure and elevated insulin levels. Having just one of these conditions contributes to your risk of serious disease, but your risk grows exponentially as the number of symptoms grows.

Visceral fat has been linked to a long list of adverse health conditions, the most serious of which are:

- High blood pressure, stroke and heart disease
- Diabetes
- Breast cancer
- Dementia

One of the main reasons visceral fat is so deadly is its role in inflammation, a natural immune response that has recently been linked to almost every chronic disease you've ever heard of. Visceral fat secretes precursors to an inflammatory chemical that helps fuel the systemic process that exacerbates early symptoms of disease.

In fact, according to a study published in *Circulation: Journal of the American Heart Association*,[2] visceral fat may have a greater impact on the cardiovascular health of older women than overall obesity. Danish researchers found that women with excessive belly fat had a greater risk of developing diseases of the arterial blood vessels than those whose fat was stored mostly in their hips, thighs and buttocks. Here's why.

▓ The proximity of visceral fat to your liver boosts production of LDL cholesterol – remember, the 'L' for 'lousy' kind – which collects in your arteries and forms plaque, a waxy substance.

▓ Over time, this waxy plaque becomes inflamed, causing swelling that narrows the arteries, restricting the passage of blood.

▓ The narrowing passageways increase blood pressure, straining your heart and potentially damaging tiny capillaries.

▓ The inflammation further increases your risk of blood clots, which can break loose and cause stroke.

How Fat Cells Work

A fat cell is like a tiny, expandable capsule – so tiny, it can only hold a microscopic drop of fat. But fat cells prefer not to live alone; they cluster together like little gangs to become fatty tissue. They generally just chill out until they're called into action by precise biochemical signals, usually hormones and enzymes. When hormones and enzymes signal fat cells, they become active, releasing fat into the bloodstream to be used for different purposes.

When you overeat, those extra calories will travel right back into those deflated fat cells and fill them back up. No matter how much weight you lose or how many hours you spend in your spinning class, your fat cells will never disappear. A deflated balloon is still a balloon.

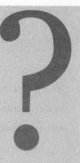
But it gets worse. Visceral fat also contributes to insulin resistance, an early precursor to diabetes. Insulin resistance is a condition in which cells do not respond to insulin and the pancreas is forced to increase production to clear the bloodstream of glucose. Over time, insulin resistance can lead to full-blown diabetes, which can severely compromise the whole circulatory system and cause long-term issues with vision, memory and wound healing.

As if that weren't enough, a study by the US-managed care organization Kaiser Permanente, comparing people with different levels of abdominal fat, showed that those who had the *most* abdominal fat were 145 per cent more likely to develop dementia, compared with people with the least amount of abdominal fat.[4] Why? Inflammation again, suggest researchers.

The One Number You Need to Remember

THE NATIONAL INSTITUTE FOR HEALTH AND CLINICAL EXCELLENCE (NICE) has stated that a waist measurement of above 35 inches for women and 40 inches for men – *no matter how much you actually weigh* – is an unhealthy sign of excess visceral fat.[5]

A measurement that specifically reflects the concentration of fat around your belly is the waist-to-hip ratio, as opposed to measuring around your hips or thighs. In other words, it's just slightly more targeted to belly fat.

Analysing data from 27,000 people in 52 countries, scientists found that heart attack sufferers had BMIs similar to, but waist-to-hip ratios higher than, those who'd never had a heart attack. Which number would you rather track?

The waist-to-hip ratio compares the measurement of the narrowest part of your waist to the broadest section of your hips. Your waist measurement should be taken in the spot that falls between the ribcage and the hip bone, as viewed from the front.

Your hip measurement is truest if you turn sideways to the mirror and make sure you incorporate your derrière in the measurement. Now divide your waist measurement by your hip measurement. For example, a woman with a 30-inch waist and 37-inch hips has a waist/hip ratio of 0.81.

According to researchers, a healthy waist-to-hip ratio for women should not exceed 0.8.[6]

Other Ways to Measure Visceral Fat

PEOPLE CAN HAVE high amounts of visceral fat despite being at a normal weight because most of that fat is stored around the abdominal organs. This understanding is relatively new and describes those who are thin on the

The Benefits of Fat

From 2 to 5 per cent of a man's body weight comes from essential fat, whereas for women, it's 10 to 13 per cent. Fat is essential in humans for:

- Energy
- Maintaining proper hormone levels
- Regulating body temperature
- Protecting vital organs
- Fertility
- Bone growth

Body fat only becomes a problem when there's too much of it. At that point, it puts a strain on your heart and other organs and starts to interfere with your body confidence.

outside but have excess fat on the inside. It's hard to imagine that one could be thin and fat at the same time, but Dr Jimmy Bell, a professor of molecular imaging at Imperial College, London, has shown that it is possible.[8] Dr Bell and his team have been using magnetic resonance imaging (MRI) machines to scan nearly 800 people in an effort to produce what they call 'fat maps'. His findings will surprise you: about 45 per cent of the thin women and 65 per cent of the slim men he tested carried excess visceral fat.

As we understand more about the dangers of visceral fat, researchers are developing increasingly more accurate – and expensive – ways to measure it. The latest test, as we go to press with this book, is one that detects levels of a protein called RBP4 (retinol binding protein 4), which is produced in higher quantities in visceral fat, compared with subcutaneous fat. In overweight people, blood levels of RBP4 are double or triple the amount found in normal-weight people. But other tests are also used, including:

BIOELECTRICAL IMPEDANCE ANALYSIS

BIOELECTRICAL IMPEDANCE ANALYSIS (BIA) is portable, easy to use and low-cost, compared with other procedures. A BIA involves circulating a very faint electrical current through the body. A device then calculates the resistance the current encounters as it travels through the body, computing body fat percentage based on height, weight and speed of the current. A faster current translates to a lower body fat percentage because electricity travels faster through muscle (a greater percentage of water is found in muscle) than it does through fat.

SONOGRAM/ULTRASOUND

ULTRASOUND MACHINES SEND out high-frequency sound waves that reflect off body structures of different densities to create a picture called a sonogram. There is no radiation exposure with this test. A clear, water-based conducting gel is applied to the skin over the area being examined to improve the transmission of the sound waves. The ultrasound transducer (a handheld probe) is then moved over the abdomen to produce an image of what's inside.

DEXA

DUAL-ENERGY X-RAY ABSORPTIOMETRY (DEXA) uses less radiation than a CT scan to assess visceral fat and is less expensive. It's typically used to assess bone mineral density but can also be a valuable tool in assessing body composition.

MRI

MAGNETIC RESONANCE IMAGING (MRI) uses powerful magnets and radio waves to create pictures without the use of radiation. Images generated by

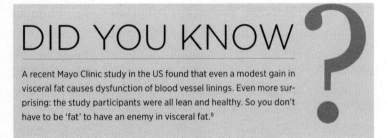

DID YOU KNOW ?

A recent Mayo Clinic study in the US found that even a modest gain in visceral fat causes dysfunction of blood vessel linings. Even more surprising: the study participants were all lean and healthy. So you don't have to be 'fat' to have an enemy in visceral fat.[9]

MRI are generally superior to – but also generally more expensive than – computed tomagraphy (see next page) because they are more finely detailed.

CT (CAT) Scan

A COMPUTED TOMOGRAPHY (CT) scanner uses radiation to create cross-sectional pictures of the body. The image results in a cross section of your belly that shows very clearly how much fat surrounds your organs. The latest scanners can image a whole body in less than 30 seconds.

Beyond Your Belly

REMEMBER, BY USING an inexpensive tape measure, you can most easily determine if your belly is endangering your health. But even if your belly measurement doesn't indicate a health risk, other things may motivate you to lose weight. Any reason is valid. No matter how or why your belly fat developed, you are clearly eager to get rid of it – and to keep it off! I'm going to offer you one of the best reasons – besides protecting your health – for trying this plan: the food! In the next chapter, you'll learn about the secret ingredients that make the *Flat Belly Diet* effective and delicious. These secret ingredients are called MUFAs.

READ A FLAT BELLY
SUCCESS
STORY

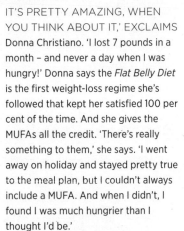

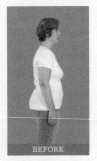
BEFORE

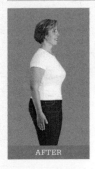
AFTER

Donna Christiano

AGE: 47

POUNDS LOST:

7

IN 32 DAYS

ALL-OVER INCHES LOST:

6.5

IT'S PRETTY AMAZING, WHEN YOU THINK ABOUT IT,' EXCLAIMS Donna Christiano. 'I lost 7 pounds in a month – and never a day when I was hungry!' Donna says the *Flat Belly Diet* is the first weight-loss regime she's followed that kept her satisfied 100 per cent of the time. And she gives the MUFAs all the credit. 'There's really something to them,' she says. 'I went away on holiday and stayed pretty true to the meal plan, but I couldn't always include a MUFA. And when I didn't, I found I was much hungrier than I thought I'd be.'

But there's more, she adds. Since she started on this plan, she's become increasingly interested in doing what is good for her. In particular, she's much more conscious of eating healthy foods. She ate healthy food before but supplemented it with a lot of junk. On one of her earlier diets, she explains, foods were assigned a certain number of points, and she'd 'spend' 15 on junk and 7 on what was good for her.

Not any more. 'I'm 47,' she says. 'I'm not getting any younger. This is the age when things start creeping up on you. So, for example, I used to love milk chocolate. Now I've started eating only dark chocolate. I try to optimize what I'm eating, too. Before, I put powdered whitener in my coffee, but now I realize that it's full of chemicals, so I've started using sweetened soya milk. I put cinnamon in coffee because it's another antioxidant. I add blueberries to my yogurt in an effort to get the most benefit I can from it.'

The best part, though, is that her belly is getting flatter. She relates a single anecdote to illustrate her success: she attended an exercise class with her neighbour Roseanne, whom she describes as tiny, tiny and *tiny*. 'She has a tiny waist, tiny hips. Just gorgeous. So we were in this class together, following along with the instructor, and I happened to glance in the mirror. I saw this woman with a really flat belly and I thought, "Oh, that's Roseanne behind me." Then I looked again. And I said to myself, "Wait a minute! That person's wearing a red shirt. *I'm* wearing a red shirt. I think that's me!"' And it *was*.

'This diet just works for me,' she raves. 'Everything about it. I'm a snacker, and I like to eat every 4 hours. That's part of the diet. I love peanut butter for breakfast, and I can have 2 tablespoons. Two tablespoons! It's practically *sliding* off the bread and I think, "Wow! This is so much food!" And the Snack Pack? Come *on*! Choco-late chips with 170g (6oz) of low-fat yogurt and a piece of fruit? Chocolate chips *on a diet*. Can you imagine?'

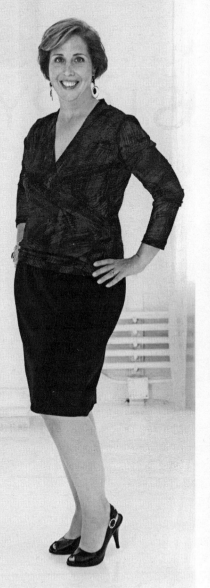

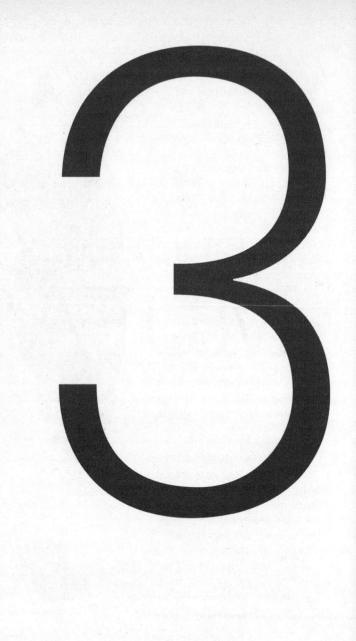

THE MAGIC OF
MUFAS

BELLY FAT MAY BE one of the most dangerous types of fat in the body, but I'm here to tell you that you don't have to live with it. You don't need to spend another day agonizing over your waistline and worrying about your rising disease risk, because there is an antidote to belly fat: MUFAs, otherwise known as monounsaturated fatty acids. There are five categories of MUFAs.

1. OILS
2. OLIVES
3. NUTS AND SEEDS
4. AVOCADOS
5. DARK CHOCOLATE

These miraculous foods hold the power to transform your body and your life. How? It's all in the name.

'MUFA' stands for **m**ono**u**nsaturated **f**atty **a**cid – a mouthful, I know – but to nutritionists like Cynthia, that mumbo jumbo perfectly describes why these plant-based fats are so healthy. Fatty acids are essentially the building blocks of all dietary fats, and like all organic elements, they're composed of atoms of carbon, oxygen and hydrogen, all lined up in a particular way to form a chain. The term *saturated* is used when every one of the carbon atoms in the chain is bound to a hydrogen atom. This makes them solid or waxy at room temperature; in your body, they're sticky and inflexible. An *unsaturated* fat is one that isn't so tightly constructed and is therefore more flexible – this flexibility is the reason that unsaturated fats are 'good' and saturated fats are 'bad'.

Think of saturated fats as sticks and unsaturated fats as strings. As saturated fats travel through your arteries, they bump and grind their way through, often getting stuck along the way. A recent study published in the *Journal of the American College of Cardiology* found that eating a meal high in saturated fat actually reduced the ability of blood vessels to expand and impaired blood flow.[1] This effect occurred just 3 hours after eating. Likewise, numerous studies have linked a long-term high intake of saturated fat to an increased risk of atherosclerosis (hardening of the arteries), heart disease, stroke and other chronic diseases.

Since MUFAs are *un*saturated (i.e. more flexible), they can easily glide through your bloodstream without gumming up the works. This flexibility is just one reason why MUFAs are so healthy; a growing body of research indicates they may actually help to unclog and protect arteries from build-up.

MUFAs Make It Big

To REALLY UNDERSTAND how MUFAs rose to nutritional stardom and why 'a MUFA at every meal' is such an important part of the *Flat Belly Diet*, I have to take you on a brief journey of the history of MUFAs. Once upon a time, in the not-so-distant past, all fats were sort of lumped together as being bad or fattening.

Recommendations from health professionals and the government based on the relationship between fats and heart disease were first introduced in the 1950s.[2] Ever since then, the emphasis has been on lowering saturated fat specifically, and the overall message has been to reduce our total fat intake. One of the long-term goals of the UK National Advisory Committee on Nutrition Education (NACNE) working party that published a discussion paper on nutritional guidelines in 1983[3] was to choose a low-fat diet that provides 'no more than 30 per cent of total food energy from fat'.

This emphasis on total fat and the 'less than 30 per cent' wording left many people thinking 'the less the better', creating scores of fat-phobic consumers who shunned not only butter and fatty meats but also vegetable oils, nuts and peanut butter. This was a constant source of frustration for experts such as Cynthia, who knew about the dangers of cutting fat too low and had studied the health benefits of plant-based oils.

More recent dietary guidelines were slightly less restrictive. In 1994 the Committee on Medical Aspects of Food Policy (COMA) published 'Nutritional Aspects of Cardiovascular Disease' following a review of new research. The report outlined recommendations for total fat at 35 per cent of food energy but had a specific recommendation to lower saturated fat to less than 11 per cent of food energy.

It acknowledged the benefits of fish and plant-based fats, recommending that most fat intake come from polyunsaturated and monounsaturated fatty acids.[4] Cynthia practically did cartwheels when she read this, particularly because she knew there was exciting research supporting the idea that not all fats were created equal.

The 'Eat Less Fat' Backlash

STUDIES FROM THE 1950s to 1970s had indicated that a high total fat intake was associated with a greater risk of cardiovascular disease (CVD). According to the British Heart Foundation, cardiovascular disease has remained the number one killer in the UK over this period. In the 1980–90s UK adults consumed over 40 per cent of their total food energy from fat.[5]

Good Fats versus Bad Fats

Dietary fat is an important energy source. Used in the production of cell membranes and certain hormones, it's critical to the regulation of blood pressure, heart rate, blood vessel constriction, blood clotting, and the nervous system. Dietary fat aids the body in absorbing vitamins such as A, D, E and K. But not all fats are created equal. Eating large amounts of the wrong fat is very hazardous to your health. But telling good fats from bad ones isn't so easy, unless you know what to look for:

THE HEALTHY

■ MONOUNSATURATED FAT (MUFA) remains liquid at room temperature but may start to solidify in the refrigerator.

■ POLYUNSATURATED FAT remains in liquid form both at room temperature and in the refrigerator. Foods high in polyunsaturated fats include vegetable oils, such as safflower, corn (maize), sunflower and soya oils.

■ OMEGA-3 FATTY ACIDS are an exceptionally healthy type of polyunsaturated fat found mostly in fat-rich seafoods such as salmon, mackerel and herring. If you'd rather do your tax return than eat two fish meals a week

The message to reduce fat intake worked – sort of. By 2000, that percentage dropped for both sexes to around 38 per cent of food energy. However, total calorie intake did not fall and the extra calories came from carbohydrates, causing the percentage of fat in the diet to shrink.

You probably remember news reports of low-fat foods from cakes to frozen yogurt flying off shelves; it was almost impossible to go food shopping without buying some sort of fat-reduced or fat-free product. With all the emphasis on fat, most people saw a green light to eat high quantities of lower-fat foods (like entire packets of reduced-fat digestives, bags of jelly beans or whole tubs of frozen yogurt). And yes, obesity prevalence rates in the UK began to skyrocket, rising in men from around 13 per cent in the early 1990s to 23 per cent in 2005 and from 16 per cent to 25 per cent for women during the same period.

(the recommended intake of healthy seafood), walnuts, flaxseeds (linseeds), flaxseed (linseed) oil and, to a lesser degree, rapeseed (canola) oil also contain omega-3 fatty acids.

THE UNHEALTHY

■ SATURATED FATS become solid or semi-solid at room temperature. The marbling in red meat is one example, as is a pat of butter. Saturated fat is found mostly in animal foods, but three vegetable sources are also high in saturated fat: coconut oil, palm (or palm kernel) oil and cocoa butter. Keep in mind that it's almost impossible to get your saturated fat intake down to zero. Even olive oil contains 2g of saturated fat per tablespoon.

■ TRANS FATS raise LDL cholesterol and lower HDL cholesterol, increasing the risk of heart disease. They're quite possibly the most hated fats in all of fatdom. Created when manufacturers hydrogenate liquid oils to increase their shelf life, they're found mostly in packaged products and nearly every food that contains shortening (or hydrogenated vegetable fat such as Trex). Look out for the words 'hydrogenated' or 'partially hydrogenated' on ingredients lists to locate – and avoid – deadly trans fats.

'Good' Fats to the Rescue

CLEARLY, THE 'EAT LESS FAT' message wasn't the answer, and in the 1990s, scientists started to pay attention to the theory that eating moderate amounts of some types of fats could actually be protective, an idea first proposed by a University of Minnesota scientist named Dr Ancel Keys, in his report called the Seven Countries Study.[6]

Between 1958 and 1970, Keys followed populations of men aged 40 to 59 in 18 areas of seven countries (US, Japan, Italy, Greece, the Netherlands, Finland and Yugoslavia). His study looked at the men's diets, disease risk factors (such as blood cholesterol levels and blood pressure) and disease rates. It was the first to look at the links between diets and disease outcomes in different populations. The study was so important because it demonstrated the degree to which the composition of the diet could predict rates of coronary heart disease. The major conclusion was that – in fact – a high fat intake was *not* associated with higher rates of heart disease.

An area that stood out was Crete, the largest of the Greek islands. Cretan men had the lowest rates of heart disease of all populations observed in the Seven Countries Study, as well as the highest average life span, despite consuming 37 per cent of their calories from fat (Finland and the US had the highest number of deaths from heart disease). Throughout the study, Keys observed that the Cretans' diets were consistent. They consumed the same types of traditional Greek meals they had been enjoying for centuries, including lots of fruit, vegetables (especially greens), nuts, beans, fish, moderate amounts of wine and cheese, small quantities of grass-fed meat, milk, eggs, some whole grains and plenty of MUFA-rich olive oil and olives. Cretan people consume on average 25 litres (44 pints) of olive oil per person each year.

Viva la Olive Oil!

THE FASCINATING FINDINGS in Crete put olive oil centre stage, and finally, the idea that some fats are healthy began to gain acceptance. Dozens of Mediterranean diet studies focusing on olive oil followed, with amazing conclusions. A Greek study concluded that the exclusive use of olive oil was associated with a 47 per cent lower likelihood of having cardiovascular disease, even after adjustments were made to account for BMI, smoking, physical activity level, educational status, a family history of heart disease, high blood pressure, high cholesterol and diabetes.[7] Another published in the *American Journal of Clinical Nutrition* in the late 1990s looked at the effects of long-term olive oil intake and blood triglyceride levels on a group of healthy men.[8] The olive oil group had significantly reduced levels of LDL cholesterol.

Numerous controlled studies have found that olive oil can lower circulating LDL levels, or prevent cholesterol from hardening. That's critical, because hardening is the beginning of the domino effect that results in artery damage and disease. But as more and more studies were conducted, it became clear that while olive oil is amazingly healthy, a great deal of its protective power lies in its MUFAs, which are also found in other plant fats, including nuts and avocado.

Eventually, research began to shift from olive oil to MUFAs and led to findings that MUFA protection extends far beyond cholesterol and heart disease. MUFAs have now been linked to reduced rates of type 2 diabetes, metabolic syndrome, breast cancer and inflammation, plus healthier blood pressure, brain function, lung function, body weight and – you guessed it – belly fat. In fact, when Cynthia showed me the pile of published studies on MUFAs specifically, I could hardly believe my eyes – it was at least as thick as this whole book. So in the interest of not overwhelming you (and saving a few trees), I've included a few of the most compelling studies. I think this summary will help you see why we're so over the moon about MUFAs.

MUFAs Protect Your Heart

▓ French scientists tested the effects of replacing some dietary carbohydrates with MUFAs without reducing calories. They found that the

MUFA-rich diet produced better effects on blood triglyceride levels and other markers for cardiovascular disease.[9]

■ Johns Hopkins researchers in the US compared the effects of three healthy diets, each with reduced saturated fat intake, on blood pressure and blood fat levels over 6 weeks, without allowing for weight loss.[10] The first diet was rich in carbohydrates, the second high in protein (with about half from plant sources) and the third high in MUFAS. They found that the protein and MUFA diets further lowered blood pressure, improved blood fat levels and reduced the estimated risk of cardiovascular disease.

■ Pennsylvania State University faculty in the US compared the cardio-vascular disease risk profile of an average American diet to four different cholesterol-lowering diets: an American Heart Association/National Cholesterol Education Program Step II diet and three high-MUFA diets.[11] The Step II diet and all of the high-MUFA diets lowered total cholesterol by 10 per cent and LDL cholesterol by 14 per cent. The MUFA diets also lowered triglyceride concentrations by 13 per cent (while the Step II increased them by 11 per cent) and did not lower 'good' HDL cholesterol (the Step II diet lowered HDL by 4 per cent).

■ University of Barcelona scientists in Spain compared the short-term effects of two Mediterranean diets versus a low-fat diet on markers of cardiovascular risk.[12] Compared with the low-fat diet, the mean changes in blood sugar, blood pressure and cholesterol were significantly better in both the MUFA-rich olive oil-based Mediterranean diet and the MUFA-rich, nut-based Mediterranean groups.

The research on MUFAs and heart health is so compelling that in many countries a daily MUFA target has now become part of the standard scientific protocol for preventing and managing cardiovascular disease risk. At present in the UK MUFA recommendations are generally calculated by the difference at a level of around 12 per cent of total food energy once saturates and polyunsaturates have been accounted for. Nevertheless, the advantages of MUFA are recognized to be of potential long-term benefit and guidelines do recommend partial replacement of saturates with MUFA.

MUFAs Ward Off Type 2 Diabetes

▓ Spanish researchers studied the effects of three weight-maintenance diets on carbohydrate and fat metabolism and insulin levels in overweight subjects by randomly assigning them to 28-day diets high in either saturated fat, monounsaturated fat (MUFAs) or carbohydrate.[13] Fasting blood sugar levels fell on both the MUFA-rich and carb-rich diets, but the MUFA diet also improved insulin sensitivity and boosted HDL cholesterol levels.

▓ At Indiana University in the US, scientists treated type 2 diabetes patients with either a MUFA-rich weight-reducing diet and or a low-fat, high-carbohydrate weight-loss diet for a 6-week period.[14] Both groups lost weight, but the MUFA group had a greater decrease in total cholesterol and triglyceride levels and a smaller drop in HDL cholesterol – and those results were sustained even after the group was allowed to regain the weight.

MUFAs Cut Metabolic Syndrome Risk

▓ Researchers from the department of medicine at Columbia University in New York studied 52 men and 33 women with metabolic syndrome (defined as any combination of low HDL cholesterol, high triglycerides or high insulin).[15] Over 7 weeks they were randomly assigned to either a typical Western diet with 36 per cent of calories from fat or two additional diets, in which 7 per cent of the calories from saturated fat were replaced with either carbohydrate or MUFAs. They found that LDL cholesterol was reduced with both the lower-saturated-fat diets, but MUFAs protected the HDL and lowered triglycerides, which were significantly higher with the high-carbohydrate diet.

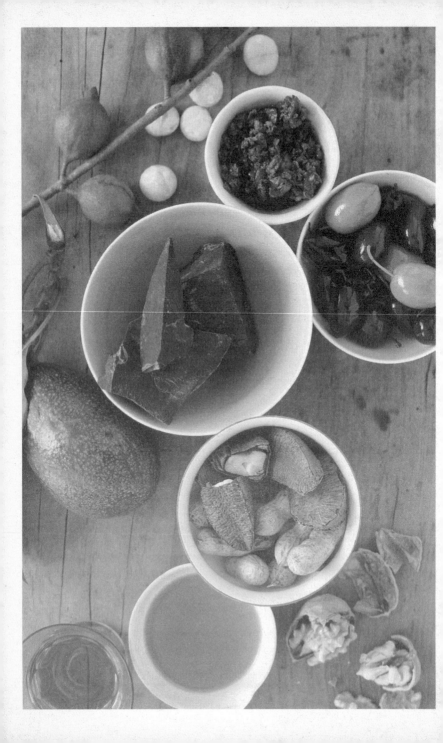

CHOOSE YOUR MUFA

These marvellous monounsaturated fat-packed foods can help you live a long, healthy life with less belly fat. But these foods also provide a host of other beneficial nutrients.

1. Oils: The health benefits of the *Flat Belly Diet*-recommended oils (canola/rapeseed, safflower, sesame, soya bean, walnut, flaxseed/linseed, sunflower, olive and peanut/groundnut) differ depending on the nut, seed or fruit they were pressed from. Flaxseed (linseed) and walnut oil are both rich sources of alpha-linolenic acid, which your body converts into omega-3 fatty acids. Extra virgin olive oil has strong antibacterial properties and can even kill *H. pylori,* the bacterium that causes most peptic ulcers and some types of stomach cancer.[16] In addition, olive oil contains phytochemicals called polyphenols, which also help prevent cardiovascular disease and cancer and reduce inflammation in the body. Canola (rapeseed), sesame, sunflower and safflower oils are all rich in vitamin E.

2. Olives: In addition to their MUFAs, olives are a good source of iron, vitamin E, copper (a mineral that protects your nerves, thyroid and connective tissue) and fibre (to regulate your digestive system, help control blood sugar levels and manage blood cholesterol).

3. Nuts and Seeds: Like oils, the health benefits of the Flat Belly nuts and seeds are numerous and varied. Sunflower seeds are a good source of linoleic acid. In a recent study, women who had the highest intakes of linoleic acid had a 23 per cent lower risk of heart disease, compared with those with the lowest intakes.[17] The omega-3 fatty acids in walnuts have been linked to protection against inflammation, heart disease, asthma and arthritis and improved cognitive function. And pistachios have been shown to help keep blood pressure down in stressful situations. Overall, nuts and seeds are good sources of many key nutrients, including protein, fibre, iron, zinc, magnesium, copper, B vitamins and vitamin E.

4. Avocados: Avocados are packed with lutein, which may help maintain healthy eyes, as well as beta-sitosterol, a natural plant sterol that may help keep cholesterol down. Adding avocado to salads and salsas has been shown to more than double the absorption of carotenoids, antioxidants linked to lower risk of heart disease and macular degeneration, a leading cause of blindness.[18] Avocados are also rich in fibre, vitamin K (which helps clot blood), potassium (which regulates blood pressure) and heart-protective folate.

5. Dark Chocolate: Dark chocolate is rich in flavanols and proanthocyanins, both of which boost good HDL cholesterol levels. It also contains natural substances that help control insulin levels and relax blood vessels, lowering blood pressure, and provides important minerals including copper, magnesium, potassium, calcium and iron.

MUFAs Reduce Inflammation

IN A NUTSHELL, inflammation is our immune system's response to stress, injury, or illness. It's a known trigger for premature ageing and disease, but MUFAs are effective at quelling its 'flames'.

■ A Spanish study focused on a large group of men and women at high risk of cardiovascular disease.[19] It found that the consumption of particular Mediterranean foods, including MUFA-rich virgin olive oil and nuts, was associated with lower blood concentrations of inflammatory markers.

■ An Italian study looked at the effect of a Mediterranean-style diet on inflammatory markers in patients with metabolic syndrome.[20] Over 3 years, researchers randomly assigned nearly 200 men and women with metabolic syndrome to either a Mediterranean-style diet rich in whole grains, fruits, vegetables and MUFA-rich nuts and olive oil, or a 'prudent' diet composed of 50 to 60 per cent carbohydrate, 15 to 20 per cent protein and 30 per cent or less fat. After 2 years, patients following the Mediterranean-style diet, who had consumed more total grams of MUFA and fibre per day, had a greater decrease in mean body weight. The high-MUFA diet also significantly reduced blood concentrations of inflammatory markers and decreased insulin resistance.

MUFAs Lower Your Risk of Breast Cancer

■ In a study published in the journal *Archives of Internal Medicine*, scientists from the department of medical epidemiology at the Karolinska Institute in Stockholm, Sweden, looked at data on 61,471 women aged 40 to 76 years from two counties in central Sweden who did not have any previous diagnosis of breast cancer.[21] After following the women over time and evaluating both their diets and incidence of breast cancer, they found an inverse association between MUFAs and breast cancer risk. There was a 45 per cent reduction in the risk of developing breast cancer for each 10-gram increment of MUFA consumed daily.

MUFAs Keep Your Brain Healthy

■ Scientists in the department of geriatrics at the Centre for the Ageing Brain at the University of Bari in Italy set out to study the relationship between diet and age-related changes in cognitive functions. The researchers looked at a sample of 5,632 people between the ages of 65 and 84 in eight regions of Italy.[22] They used a battery of standardized tests to assess cognitive function, selective attention and memory, evaluated the subjects' diets and found that those with the highest percentage of calories from MUFAs had the greatest protection against cognitive decline.

■ Another Italian study, led by scientists at the centre's Memory Unit, investigated the role of diet in age-related cognitive decline (ARCD) by studying an elderly population in southern Italy that consumed a typical Mediterranean diet.[23] They also concluded that high intake of MUFAs warded off ARCD.

MUFAs Extend Your Life

■ Several studies have looked at the link between MUFA intake and life expectancy. An 8½-year follow-up to the Italian Longitudinal Study on Ageing investigated the possible role of MUFAs and other foods in protecting against death from any cause.[24] Among subjects without dementia between the ages of 65 and 84, scientists found that a higher MUFA intake was associated with an increase of survival, and there was no effect found in any other selected food group.

MUFAs Target Belly Fat

■ A 2007 study published in the US journal *Diabetes Care* found that a MUFA-rich diet prevented central body fat distribution, compared with a high-carbohydrate and high-saturated-fat diet of the same calorie level.[25]

■ Australian researchers randomly assigned overweight men to various 4-week diets composed of the same calorie level with different amounts of saturated, monounsaturated and polyunsaturated fat. The MUFA-rich diet resulted in lower total body weight and body fat. The authors concluded that a high-MUFA diet can induce a significant loss of body weight and fat mass without a change in total calorie or fat intake.

■ Another Aussie study compared post-meal body fat-burning rates after two breakfasts: one with saturated fat from cream and one with MUFA from olive oil.[26] The MUFA group had a significantly higher fat-burning rate in the 5 hours following the MUFA breakfast, particularly in the subjects with greater abdominal fat.

The Other Antidote to Belly Fat: Attitude

OF COURSE, THE *Flat Belly Diet* isn't only about food. Before we get to the eating plan, I want you to understand the one factor that will be key to making your dream of a flat belly come true – and that's your state of mind. Your emotions, stress level and body image all play a role in how and when you eat – and even how and where you put on weight. That's right – your emotional state can actually cause you to store belly fat. In the next chapter, we'll explore this mind–belly connection in depth and reveal the secret to succeeding on the *Flat Belly Diet*. But for now, let's bask in the glorious knowledge that flattening your belly may be as easy as drizzling olive oil on your next salad, spreading peanut butter on a cracker or – oh, yes – licking melted chocolate off your fingertips.

READ A FLAT BELLY
SUCCESS
STORY

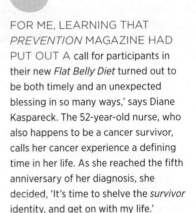

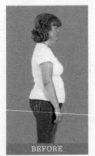

BEFORE

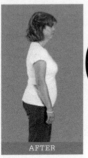

AFTER

Diane Kaspareck

AGE: 52

POUNDS LOST:

6.5
IN 32 DAYS

ALL-OVER INCHES LOST:

6.25

FOR ME, LEARNING THAT *PREVENTION* MAGAZINE HAD PUT OUT A call for participants in their new *Flat Belly Diet* turned out to be both timely and an unexpected blessing in so many ways,' says Diane Kaspareck. The 52-year-old nurse, who also happens to be a cancer survivor, calls her cancer experience a defining time in her life. As she reached the fifth anniversary of her diagnosis, she decided, 'It's time to shelve the *survivor* identity, and get on with my life.'

Part of that decision included going on the *Flat Belly Diet*. 'It was just at that time that I heard about the diet,' she recalls, 'so I decided to give myself a 5-year anniversary gift.' Her goal was to improve her health, shed her excess weight and return her body to a complete state of balance. 'It was one of the first times in my life I had ever done anything that was *only* for me.'

The first weekend on the diet, Diane sent her husband and son off to the beach, and she stayed at home alone to concentrate on the food plan. 'I realized there is a learning curve with it, so I started very methodically, shopping for the food and making the meals and sitting down by myself to enjoy them. I decided to start walking every day, too, and it all just took off from there.

'It's interesting,' she says. 'As you start to deal with your health issues and

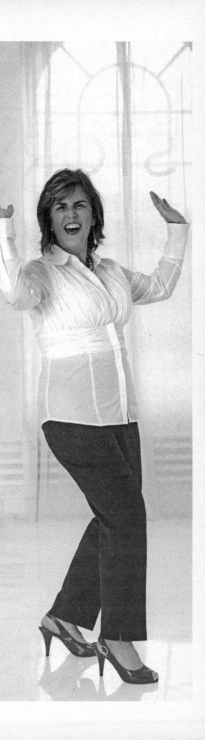

get better at it, you start treating yourself better. You connect more to yourself in a lot of different ways. Even mentally you're feeling better. Things aren't as overwhelming, maybe because you have more energy.'

She's thrilled with that new-found energy. In the past, she used to come home from work and drop onto the sofa just in time for afternoon TV. 'That was it for me – I was done for the evening. I was tired and maybe even a little bit depressed.' Things are different now. The food she's eating and the weight loss have energized her. She's out in the evenings and wanting to do more and more. 'It's as if I have got back another 6 hours a day of my life,' she says.

'I know it's just a diet, but I feel so good. And I'm so much happier. Cancer takes away some of your control, but now I feel as though I have a handle on a controllable issue. My body is in a really good equilibrium as far as nutrition goes, and I feel calmer and more relaxed – like nothing scary is going to jump out of the wardrobe at me.'

Diane lost only 6½lb on the first 32 days of the *Flat Belly Diet*, but her muscle mass and her body fat percentage changed. She feels losing slowly is a good thing. 'Do I want to lose more? Of course,' she says. 'But I realized in the big picture, that's just how it is. You don't gain it or lose it overnight. I really feel as though I've got some fabulous new habits that will stay with me. And I'm going to keep going until I lose every pound I set out to lose.'

4

THE MIND–BELLY CONNECTION

THE RELATIONSHIP BETWEEN mind and body is pretty solid. Understanding how they work together is key to reaching your weight loss – or any – lifestyle goal. Why? Consider the role your emotions, attitudes and feelings play in what you eat, how much you eat and when you eat it.

I clearly recall the day it dawned on me that my relationship to food is profoundly affected by my body image. It was back in the 1980s, and it was all about a mirror. I had just moved into my first apartment and, needing to give myself the once-over and ensure that my skirt wasn't tucked into my tights before heading out each day, I bought a full-length mirror and propped it against a wall.

For the next month, I smiled happily at the longer, leaner image I saw every morning. Wondering if I'd magically lost a few pounds on move-in day, I weighed myself on the scales at the gym. No, hadn't lost anything. But goodness, did I feel thinner! I was so motivated by this state of affairs that over the next couple of weeks, I decided to maintain the healthy momentum. I ran further, ate smaller portions, skipped desserts and took fewer handfuls from the office sweetie bowl.

Then I finally got around to hanging the mirror properly. That's when I discovered that tilting a mirror against a wall (with the bottom of the glass closer to you than the top) makes your reflection appear longer and leaner. When I hung that mirror flush against the wall and turned to see my profile, I came face-to-face with reality. What I saw was hardly 'fat' – just slightly less *flat*. Still, it was a major blow to my body confidence. I drove straight to McDonald's and ordered a Big Mac®. True story.

Years of experience of talking to women who have tried many diets shows that attitude, emotions, thoughts, feelings and practically everything mind-related all influence the foods you choose to eat and the way you eat them. That's why the *Flat Belly Diet* is about engaging your mind as much as your tastebuds. Only if your brain is on board will you enjoy success.

Conquer Emotional Eating

PHYSIOLOGICALLY SPEAKING, your appetite is controlled by biochemical signals that tell your brain that you're hungry and need to eat or satisfied and can stop. The problem is, we've all learned to override those signals. We eat not only when we're hungry but also when we're happy or sad, relaxed or anxious.

To get a handle on emotional eating, you need to understand why you do it. For one thing, many of us have been conditioned to believe that food can bring comfort (remember getting a lollipop after an injection at the doctor's?). And it does, at least in the short term. As adults, many of us turn to food to relieve feelings of stress. Snacking is a common response to boredom, anxiety, anger and, yes, loneliness. (I've been known to rely on spoonfuls of peanut butter when faced with writer's block.)

For many of us, years of eating to address everything *but* an empty stomach means we have to relearn what actual hunger feels like. Although we often don't recognize it, the line between emotional hunger and *true* hunger is actually quite clear. US research has identified five ways to differentiate between the two:[1]

1. Emotional hunger comes on suddenly, while physical hunger is gradual.

2. Physical hunger is felt below the neck (growling stomach), while emotional hunger is felt above the neck (a craving for ice cream).

3. When only a certain food like pizza or chocolate will meet your need, your 'hunger' is born of emotion. When your body requires fuel, you're more open to other food options.

4. Emotional hunger wants to be satisfied instantly. Physical hunger can wait.

5. Emotional hunger leaves guilt in its wake. Physical hunger doesn't.

Recognizing these signals can help you distinguish an emotional need for food from a physical one. The next time a craving strikes, try this: ignore the signals coming from the neck up. Are you physically hungry? Ask yourself what you're feeling emotionally and how you can meet these mental (versus physical) needs.

The real cure for emotional eating is developing effective coping strategies, not just seeking out distractions. Here's an example: when you're sad and craving ice cream, cleaning out your cupboards may direct you away from the freezer, but it won't help you exorcise that melancholy feeling. Too often, we fail to take the very important steps of first identifying the emotions we're experiencing and, second, *feeling* them. If you're feeling sad, watch a tearjerker and allow yourself to have a good cry. Or phone a close friend who's good at listening at such times. Addressing the emotion rather than avoiding it is the best way to release yourself from the desire to eat.

Address the Stress Factor

WHEN SCIENTISTS STUDY STRESS, they always differentiate between two types: *acute* or short-term, and *chronic* or long-term. An example of *chronic* stress could be having a job you dislike but feel you can't escape from. An example of short-term or *acute* stress? It might be as ordinary as being late for a meeting or as life-threatening as almost being hit by a car.

Back in the Stone Age, our species' very survival depended on the ability to respond instantly to short-term stresses like being chased by predators. Today, we're still equipped with a hair-trigger mechanism that overrides our rational minds in an emergency or when we feel threatened. We call it the fight-or-flight response, and it's no different if the stressor is a ravenous beast or an impatient boss. Here's how it works.

THE BIOLOGY OF ACUTE STRESS

STRESS RESPONSES BEGIN in the nervous system. The central nervous system (CNS) responds to orders from the conscious mind, while the autonomic nervous system (ANS) functions independently. If you decide, for example, to take a picture of a friend with your mobile phone, the CNS puts into play all the actions involved in completing the task, from having the idea to taking the picture. Meanwhile, you will continue to breathe (without having to think about it), and your body will continue to go about the business of digesting food, pumping blood and fending off harmful bacteria.

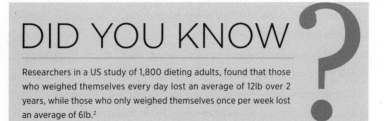

DID YOU KNOW

Researchers in a US study of 1,800 dieting adults, found that those who weighed themselves every day lost an average of 12lb over 2 years, while those who only weighed themselves once per week lost an average of 6lb.[2]

Your ANS governs these functions, operating without a single conscious
thought or action on your part.

Within the ANS, there are two branches: the sympathetic nervous system
(SNS) and the parasympathetic nervous system (PNS). The first revs you up,
and the second calms you down. Say, for example, you're crossing a busy
road and see an out-of-control car heading straight for you. You don't con-
sciously order your heart to pump faster and deliver more blood to your
muscles so they can react with more force to get you out of the way; you just
naturally jump onto the kerb. In that mere millisecond, your brain perceives
the threat and kicks the SNS into high gear. Here's what happens next.

■ The hypothalamus in the brain sends a message to your adrenal glands
near your kidneys, which pump out the hormones adrenalin and cortisol
(more on this later).

■ Adrenalin increases your heartbeat to twice its normal speed, send-
ing extra blood to the brain, as well as to the major muscles in your
arms and legs – so you're better able to dodge that moving car.

■ Your memory gets sharper.

■ Your immune system goes on alert – in case it's needed to fight infec-
tion from an impending wound.

■ Your arteries narrow – so if you're injured, you'll lose less blood.

■ Narrowed arteries cause an increase in blood pressure.

- Your pupils dilate and your vision becomes more acute.
- Your digestive system slows down.
- Insulin production ramps up, overriding signals from adrenalin to burn fat and encourages the body to store it in anticipation of future needs.

All this happens to get you safely out of the way of that car hurtling towards you – and, once upon a time, to enable our ancestors to dodge that hungry sabre-toothed tiger intent on landing its next meal. When the immediate threat is over, so is the short-term stress. That's when the PNS steps in, releasing calming hormones and your body returns once again to equilibrium.

THE HIGH PRICE OF CHRONIC STRESS

UNLIKE ACUTE STRESS, which has a beginning and an end, chronic stress is ongoing. When your marriage hits a rough patch, your child has trouble at school, you finally get that promotion and your workload doubles, your ageing parents suddenly need a lot more care – or all of these things happen at once! – that is chronic stress. The problem is, your body still reacts as if these stresses were acute, yet – and here's the important distinction – there's no calming period. The SNS just keeps doing its stuff, keeping you in a state of heightened physiological arousal as if your very life were being threatened, 24/7. The more your body's stress response system is activated, the more difficult it is to switch off. And that's a major concern, given that anywhere from 60 to 90 per cent of illness is stress-related. Here's how the stress–health connection works.

In times of stress, the adrenal glands secrete an abundance of cortisol. Normally, cortisol's role is to *regulate* blood pressure, cardiovascular function and metabolism. Your body can easily handle the occasional burst of cortisol triggered by an acute or high-stress moment – no problem there. It's when the stress is chronic and a steady stream of cortisol begins to flow into your bloodstream that things start to go bad. Too much cortisol weakens your immune system, puts your heart into overdrive and raises your blood pressure. A consistently high level of circulating stress hormones adversely affects brain function as well, especially memory. And excessive cortisol can also interfere with 'feel-good' neurotransmitters such as dopamine and serotonin, making you more vulnerable to depression.

Cortisol and Belly Fat

REST ASSURED, I haven't forgotten why you're here. This is a book about belly fat, so let's turn our attention now to cortisol and its affinity for our bellies. Research has shown that cortisol not only stimulates the appetite but also specifically induces cravings for sugar and fat – the most easily burned 'fuels'. This helps explain why many of us eat when we're stressed; it also sheds some light on why it's the tub of ice cream we reach for rather than a nice crisp apple.

Signs of Chronic Stress

- Headaches
- Frequent upset stomach, indigestion, trapped wind, diarrhoea or appetite changes
- Feeling as though you might cry
- Muscular tension
- Tightness in your chest and a feeling that you can't catch your breath
- Feeling nervous or sad
- Feeling irritable and angry
- Having problems at work or in your normal relationships
- Sleep disturbance: either insomnia or hypersomnia (sleeping too much)
- Apathy (lack of interest, motivation or energy)
- Mental or physical fatigue
- Frequent illness
- Hives or skin rashes
- Tooth grinding
- Feeling faint or dizzy
- Ringing in the ears
- Disruptions/skips in menstrual cycle; unusually severe PMS or menopausal symptoms

But here's the killer: cortisol also signals the body to *store* fat centrally, around the organs. That's right – on your belly. It's nature's way of ensuring that resources are readily and easily available for fuel when the body needs them to perform life-preserving exertion or, for that matter, withstand famine. This all makes even more sense when you take into account the fact that abdominal fat has both a greater blood supply (so cortisol travels there quickly) and more receptors for cortisol.

You *Can* Take Control!

AFTER EACH OF my life's most terrifying moments – piano recital at the age of 9, gymnastic competition at 12, first television appearance at 25 – my mother always told me, to my great surprise, that I didn't look the least bit nervous. If she only knew what was happening inside! As I've grown older, I have learned a few tried-and-true methods for managing the day-to-day pressures of running a magazine, bringing up my daughters and tackling hundreds of other projects, like writing this book. My main tactic is to heap lots of gratitude onto the world's greatest husband and best nanny. After that, I aim for regular exercise, laughing really hard at least once a day and actually saying the words 'I am so lucky to have you' to my husband, Steve, and daughters, Sophia and Olivia, whenever I can.

For me, these tactics give me focus, perspective and help me stay calm (on most days of the week!). It's easy for me to tell you to reduce stress by 'finding a hobby' or 'asking your children to do the dishes more often', but how helpful are these suggestions, really? A colleague writes in her gratitude journal every day. My husband kayaks on the quietest lake he can find. And an editor friend meditates every morning – an idea I love but an activity I just can't wrap my brain around . . . yet. (I'm working on it.) My point is: since your sources of stress are personal, so should be the ways you counteract their effects.

However, researchers have targeted certain behaviours that will be helpful for most women trying to manage busy lives, deflect anxiety and find happiness. These seven stress-busting strategies will not only help you feel calm and live a more relaxing existence but will prevent stress-induced weight gain in the process. Use this list like a tool kit. The more tools you use, the more you'll benefit.

Get Calm! 7 Stress-busting Strategies

1. GET MORE SLEEP. Diaries kept at the turn of the 20th century, before electric lighting became commonplace, show that people often slept about 9 hours a night. Can you imagine? Nowadays most of us are lucky to get 7. This doesn't just make you tired; it can make you stressed – and fat. Consistently depriving yourself of rest subjects your body to a constant level of

Not All Stress Is Harmful

Believe it or not, some kinds of acute stress are beneficial. Researchers in the US found that stress from engaging in a memory task activated the immune system, whereas the stress created by passively watching a violent video weakened immunity (as measured by salivary concentration of sIgA, a major immune factor). These results suggest that minor mental challenges and deadlines at work could help strengthen your body's defences.[5]

elevated stress. Sleep deprivation results in reduced levels of leptin, a protein that regulates body fat and increases ghrelin, which stimulates appetite. So not getting enough sleep causes your body to store fat, slows your metabolism and makes you want to eat more. Your body must have enough time to rest to revitalize and replenish its reserves. This is especially true for anyone on a diet, because if you're in any way sleep deprived, it's that much more difficult to summon the physical energy and mental focus to stick to any diet *or* exercise plan. I urge you: if you do nothing else on this list, put getting a good night's sleep at the top of your *Flat Belly* to-do list.

■ Slip on some socks. The instant warm-up provided by socks widens blood vessels and allows your body to transfer heat from its core to the extremities, cooling you slightly. This induces sleep, says Dr Phyllis Zee, director of sleep disorders at Northwestern University's Feinberg School of Medicine in the US. If you wear an old-fashioned nightcap, you can achieve the same result.[6]

■ Stick to your schedule. People who follow regular daily routines report fewer sleep problems than those with more unpredictable lifestyles, according to a study from the University of Pittsburgh Medical Center. Recurring time cues will synchronize your body rhythms and sleep–wake cycles, explains Dr Lawrence Epstein.[7]

■ Go dark. Any light will signal the brain to wake up, but 'blue light' from your mobile phone and your clock's digital display is the worst offender. Dim your clock and eliminate lighted devices from the bedroom.

2. GET SOME DISTANCE. Take note of the things that cause you chronic stress – and, when possible, sidestep them. When emotions run high, you may find yourself biting your nails, leaning on your car horn, forgetting important appointments, even yelling at your kids. If you think about what's bothering you – really think about it – you'll probably find it's not your nails or your children or the traffic that's the problem. It's that you've used up what I like to think of as your stress reserves, and you need to interrupt the stress cycle. When this happens, remove yourself from the scene. Just walk away. Literally. Go around the corner or just into the next room. If even that is impossible, simply close your eyes, count to 10 and breathe deeply. Those few simple moments might give you a chance to process strong emotions before they overwhelm you. Physically, you should feel better almost immediately.

3. GET MOVING. EVERY DAY. Studies show that even 10 minutes of physical activity will help reduce levels of cortisol in the bloodstream. Exercise changes your body's biochemistry, triggering the brain to produce beta-endorphins, chemicals that calm you down, regulate your stress hormones and make you feel good. So the next time you feel like pulling your hair out or reaching for a handful of crisps, head out of the door and take a bike ride or even just a quick walk. A little exercise may not solve the problem at hand, but it will certainly help you cope with it.

4. GET CONNECTED. Talking with others can defuse your feelings of tension, but studies have shown that even just being in someone's company – without saying a word – helps alleviate stress. It also promotes good health: research shows that people who maintain personal and community connections have better health than those who don't.

Walk for Deep Sleep

A little walking goes a long way towards getting a sound night's sleep. When researchers studied more than 700 men and women, they found that those who walked at least 1km a day at a moderate pace were one-third less likely to have sleeping problems than those who walked shorter distances. Those who walked at a brisker pace were most likely of all to enjoy sound sleep. Other studies show that a regular walking programme is as effective at improving sleep as medication.

An important caveat to keep in mind: only spend time with people who leave you energized, not emotionally drained. If there is any doubt about which is which, ask yourself this question after you've been with the person: did I have fun, or did I work hard to make sure my *friend* had fun? Of course, the answer to both of these questions can be yes, but if the answer to the first question is no, that's a pretty good clue that you need to find someone else to spend time with. Emotionally draining people – or, in the popular terminology of today, toxic people – do very little to boost your self-confidence or keep you on track towards your goals.

5. GET POSITIVE. Stop that negative self-talk. I'm referring to that little voice in your head that passes judgment on your every move. Whenever you catch yourself thinking, 'I'll never get this report done' or 'My house is a filthy mess', stop yourself and redirect your thinking. Instead, replay the thought but with a positive spin: 'I will do my absolute best to meet this deadline' and 'I love this house for all its wonderful memories'. Forcing these thoughts into your head might feel silly, but I promise you: it will help you feel more in control of your life, and it will build your self-respect and self-confidence. And, as we now know, that is integral to achieving your health and weight-loss goals!

Stop Wasting Time

A little time management can go a long way to remedy stress. Keep in mind: time management isn't necessarily about doing more – it's about doing more of the things you *want* to do. Try keeping a time tracker for a day or two to find out where your time is really going.

Set up a daily timetable on your computer or in a journal, broken into 15-minute blocks. Track what you do in each block of time from when you wake up to when you go to bed, and evaluate each day. Seeing how you actually spend your time throughout the day may help you determine how you can make small changes that reduce your stress and improve your ability to fit in healthy meals, more physical activity or just a little downtime.

*'The
Mental
Tweak
That Will
Set You Up
for Success'*

If there's one thing I've learned from my years of nutrition counselling, it's this: to make lasting changes, you've got to believe that what you're getting is much better than what you're giving up. What's worked for my clients is doing some self-exploration to arrive at a place where the pros of changing truly outweigh the cons – not because they *think* that's where they should be, but because they believe it!

I once had a client who told me she'd never understood those people who'd *really* rather have an apple and almonds than a few chocolate biscuits. She always thought they were lying or had an iron will when they'd pass on (free!) goodies at work and eat the healthy foods they'd brought instead. Then, one Monday afternoon, she was reaching for a box of chocolates when it hit her. She'd spent the last week eating healthy foods and had been able to join her family on a bike ride. For the first time in a long time, they hadn't gone without her. The satisfaction she got from that bike ride meant more than the momentary satisfaction the chocolate would provide. In that instant, she really did want a crisp apple instead of those biscuits. And her choice had nothing to do with willpower.   *– Cynthia*

6. GET CENTRED – SELF-CENTRED. Before you go any further, I want you to grab a pencil and fill in the blanks.

Below, write the names of the most important people in your life.

_____

_____

_____

_____

When you have completed your list, turn to the next page in this book. *Don't turn the page until you have completed this list.*

OK. Did you put yourself at the top of your own list? Are you even *on* your list? My guess is that if you *did* include yourself, you were at the bottom. And that's not surprising, because most women are so *other-directed* that they completely overlook their own happiness and needs. If I asked you about your relationship with your husband or your parents or your children, no doubt you could give me specific, detailed, layered answers. But if I asked you to describe how you treat yourself, how different would the answer be?

When you're trying to change a behaviour (particularly a health-orientated behaviour like eating better and exercising more), it's absolutely essential to learn to put yourself first. After all, what is a diet if not a contract between you and yourself? You have chosen to read and follow the principles of the *Flat Belly Diet*. I presume you've done this for the sake of how you look, how you feel and how your health measures up. And while you've made a commitment to stay on the food plan – it's far more than that. It's a commitment to put yourself at the top of the agenda, to recognize that you are special and you deserve the time, energy and effort that's equal to everything else in your life.

Now I want you to find a nice sheet of clean, crisp paper and rewrite the list of the most important people in your life. This time put yourself at the top, where you rightfully belong. Put the list somewhere you'll see it often, like on your mirror or the refrigerator door. You'll be amazed how much less stressful life is when you remember to always look out for Number One.

7. GET IT ON THE CALENDAR. Now that you have placed yourself at the top of the list, acknowledge that 'me' time is not an indulgence but an *essential* factor in your health and happiness, not to mention your success on the *Flat Belly Diet*. 'Me' time is yours to take, if you're willing to say, 'This is *my* moment, and it takes priority over everything else.' How about starting with 15 minutes a day?

I know what you're thinking: *I don't have 15 minutes!* You're wrong, and I'm going to prove it to you. On the first 4 days of this plan, I'm going to ask you to take 2 to 3 minutes before every meal to focus on yourself, your ultimate goal and how much you can achieve when you put your mind to it. I call these little exercises Mind Tricks because they're simple tasks that help wake up your brain and draw your attention to the act of eating. If you can manage a few minutes before every meal, you've found your 15 minutes.

SASS FROM SASS

"Just Say No to Trans Fats."

I'm a firm believer in eating fat, but in creating this plan, I was adamant that a certain type of fat should be excluded altogether: trans fatty acids, or trans fats. These man-made fats are created from vegetable oils in a process called partial hydrogenation, which adds hydrogen to liquid unsaturated oils. This changes their structure into a form that helps hold ingredients together in foods like pie crusts, biscuits or crackers. Because trans fats spoil more slowly, they extend a product's shelf life. Research shows that not only are trans fats bad for your heart because they clog arteries and raise 'bad' LDL cholesterol, but they also increase the accumulation of belly fat, according to US research. To avoid trans fats, look at all ingredients lists. If the words *hydrogenated* or *partially hydrogenated* appear, limit or avoid the food.   – Cynthia

As you continue past the 4th day on the *Flat Belly Diet*, I'll discuss the importance of keeping a journal. This will help you focus your mind and reflect on your aims, to ensure you continue to be inspired throughout the programme. Make sure you write in your journal every day so you truly keep track of your progress.

Armed and Ready: The Big Three Questions

NOW YOU UNDERSTAND the scientific underpinnings of both emotional eating and the body's physiological response to stress. And you can now master the unique forces at work in the mind–belly connection. You're also equipped with seven useful stress-busting strategies that will help you manage the stress in your life during this journey of healthy eating.

But before we embark on the first part of the *Flat Belly Diet* – the Four-Day Anti-Bloat Jumpstart – I want you to take a few moments to reflect on these three vital change-related questions.

1. *Who am I doing this for?*

   There is only one acceptable answer to this question, and that is 'me' – and no one else. You're probably a lot more comfortable doing things for others, but how often do you really do something for yourself? Losing weight, if

Why do I have to keep a food journal?

The food journal serves several functions. First, food journals raise your awareness about exactly what and how much you're eating. Research also tells us that dieters benefit from accountability, particularly when they're starting out on a new plan. Writing in a journal each day will help you stay committed to your goals, keep your behaviour on track and lead you to better results.

you need to, is really the ultimate expression of self-caring, more so than booking the occasional massage or regular manicure and pedicure. That's because losing weight now, especially if you're overweight or obese, can make the difference between feeling tired and feeling energized. It can mean the difference between a retirement you'll enjoy and one plagued by health problems like diabetes or heart disease. As I noted before, the fat in your belly is the most dangerous and deadly. Choosing to cure yourself – especially with a plan like this that promises not just weight loss but also a whole host of other health benefits – may be the greatest gift you can give yourself.

2. *How can I make the next 32 days easier?*

Think *Flat Belly* feng shui. I'm not talking about moving your fridge into the cellar or hanging a mirror over your cooker. I'm simply suggesting that you consider all the ways you can make your office and home surroundings more supportive of your new goal. That means divesting the kitchen cupboard and refrigerator of tempting food or keeping all the junk food in the second cupboard on the left. As for your office, you may want to clean out your 'junk' drawer. That 'emergency' chocolate stash isn't going to do you any favours. And now is the time to find somewhere to put your Snack Pack.

3. *Who's on My Team?*

Before you begin, consider having a serious heart-to-heart with everyone in your immediate circle. Tell them why you're doing this, why it's so important to you, what you need from them and how you think it might affect your relationship. You might need to swap your family's Sunday bacon roll stop with a healthier breakfast at home, or a drink with the girls for a cup of tea at a local café. When they realize how important this is to you, they'll listen and I'll bet some of them will even want to join in!

READ A FLAT BELLY
SUCCESS
STORY

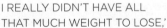

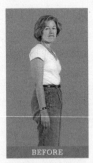

BEFORE

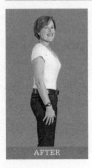

AFTER

Kathy Brechner

AGE: 53

POUNDS LOST:

5

IN 32 DAYS

ALL-OVER
INCHES LOST:

7.5

I REALLY DIDN'T HAVE ALL THAT MUCH WEIGHT TO LOSE,' Kathy Brechner says. 'Only 5 pounds, actually. But believe me, they were the *toughest* pounds I've ever tried to get off in my life.' She credited much of the difficulty in losing this weight to the fact that she's 53 and hovering near the menopause. But her lifestyle wasn't helping, either. 'I work for the local education authority, so I'm often on the run. I'm eating in the car half the time, eating late at night, not exercising enough, running the kids around to their activities in between. Something had to give.'

Kathy was concerned that 'something' would be her health because, as she points out, she has a family history of heart disease, type 2 diabetes and high blood pressure. And so, with the image in the back of her mind of the number on the scales slowly creeping up, and knowing that at this point in her life she was facing the same fate as her parents, she realized it was time to see what new steps she might take to improve on what she was already doing – particularly since what she was doing simply wasn't working.

That was when she learned about the *Flat Belly Diet* and its focus on good health as well as weight loss. She was already familiar with the benefits of eating MUFAs and the healthy style of Mediterranean-type foods. But she felt she needed more structure. 'I think that was the initial attraction,' she explains. 'I just liked the idea of the 32-day principle. I knew I could do anything for 32 days, so why not give it a try?'

She says the diet completely changed how she and her family view portions. 'My husband looked at the menu I had chosen for one of our dinners and said, *"Two tablespoons of pasta? Who can get by on 2 tablespoons of pasta?"* But we not only could – we did. For snacks, I have a flat wicker tray on the worktop, and I have small dishes of the different nuts sitting there. A measuring spoon is right next to it because it's just too easy to grab handfuls and stuff them down before you know it. The diet has even covered the "quick grab" for nights when I have meetings. I could have a prepared meal and know I was giving something healthy to my family and still sticking to the diet.'

Is she happy with her results? 'I'm ecstatic!' she says. 'The *Flat Belly Diet* brought me to the goal I set out to achieve: 5 pounds – gone. For the first time. And as a bonus, my energy level is so much higher than it's been in the past. I'm not getting any more sleep. I haven't been doing any additional exercise. So it has to be what I'm eating.' She adds, 'I think every woman at or approaching the menopause should know this: there's never a better time to start thinking about your health than *right now*. Keeping your weight down and your energy up gets harder as you age, so why not be a little ahead of that curve?'

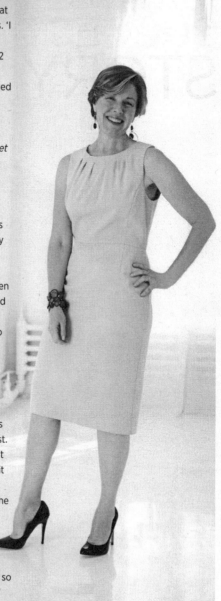

5

THE FOUR-DAY
ANTI-BLOAT
JUMPSTART

THIS CHAPTER IS A DREAM COME TRUE for any woman who's ever suffered from a bloated belly. A number of factors influence how bloated you feel on any given day, including what you eat and how you take care of yourself. But this chapter will help you address your bloating – whatever its cause – immediately. In just 4 days, you'll lose several pounds and inches, which will start a cascade of motivation and energy that will immediately set you up for success on the rest of the plan.

I was in my twenties when I first really understood the phenomenon of water retention. I was a magazine editor at the time, and every Friday morning, the staff met at 9 a.m. sharp in a big new conference room on the far side of the floor. It was in that room that I noticed that my engagement ring always seemed to mysteriously fit more snugly.

Once I noticed the connection between the mysterious swelling and a particular day and time, I started paying a little more attention to what I ate and drank the rest of the week. And then I realized what was happening: Thursday was pizza night. Every week, I'd meet my then-fiancé, Steve, for a pizza at Mama Santa's in Little Italy. *And I'd put salt on every piece.*

Bloating can really ruin a girl's day, not to mention her confidence. That's why the *Flat Belly Diet* starts with a Four-Day Anti-Bloat Jumpstart Plan. This phase will start a cascade of confidence because it promises to shrink your belly – a loss of up to $5^3/_4$ total inches – in just 4 short days. How do I know? Because we tested the entire *Flat Belly Diet* – including the Jumpstart – on women just like you, holding weigh-ins on a biweekly basis. You're reading their stories throughout this book. More than half of our test panel lost at least 1 full inch from their bellies during the Jumpstart period.

There's nothing more satisfying and confidence-boosting when you're starting a new eating plan than being able to see – almost immediately – your trousers getting looser, your cheekbones getting more noticeable, your muscles getting more defined. It inspires commitment and a desire to suc-

DID YOU KNOW ?

The word *metabolism* refers to the number of calories you burn per day. Some of that comes from the energy your cells use to perform everyday life-saving functions (like maintaining heart muscle contractions that keep your blood flowing). That's called your basal metabolic rate. You also burn calories through activity, whether that's taking out the rubbish or running a 5-K. The last piece of the metabolism puzzle comes from digesting your food, which burns calories. This is called the 'thermic effect' of food. The sum of all the calories you burn (basal + activity + digestion) equals your total metabolism, or total metabolic rate.

Being less active affects your metabolism in two ways: it makes the second 'plus' in this equation smaller, but you also lose muscle, which reduces the basal number in the equation.

ceed. And that's what I want you to get out of this book more than anything else: success.

The Four-Day Anti-Bloat Jumpstart Plan has been created for the very specific purpose of eliminating wind, heavy solids and excess fluid so you will quickly feel and look lighter. Bear in mind: this is *not* a wacky – and dangerous – 'detox' plan. You'll be eating whole fruits, vegetables and grains and fresh, naturally flavoured water – wholesome food prepared in simple, delicious ways. In fact, it's what you *won't* be eating and drinking and doing that really makes the Jumpstart so effective. To see how, I think it helps to first understand how your digestive system works.

Digestion – the basics

YOUR GASTROINTESTINAL (GI) tract is about 35 feet long from top to bottom. Read that again: *35 feet long!* That's about seven of you, lying end to end. And it's all coiled up inside your torso (along with most of your major organs and, yes, belly fat). That's why, when your GI tract is irritated or in any way dysfunctional, it greatly impacts on how you feel overall. But before we talk about potential problems, let's go over the basics.

The primary role of your GI tract is to extract essential nutrients like carbohydrates, proteins, fats, vitamins, minerals and water from the food you eat and the beverages you drink. These nutrients are transported through the walls of the small and large intestines into the bloodstream, where they're then distributed to wherever they're needed. For instance, when you eat a turkey sandwich, your GI tract breaks it down into bits of carbohydrate (the bread and vegetables), protein (the turkey), fat (the mayo), fibre (from the bread) and all sorts of vitamins and minerals. Carbohydrates, protein and fat get broken down even further into sugars, amino acids and fatty acids, respectively. The sugars go to fuel brain and muscle activity (not to mention the doings of every cell in your body), the amino acids get used to build muscle and bone and the fats get stored for future energy needs or get used to manufacture hormones and other essential compounds.

Ultimately, hundreds of biochemical reactions occur, and the chemical end products of that turkey sandwich have thousands of uses. But you can see that the ultimate job of your digestive system is to extract as much nutrition as possible out of everything you put in your mouth.

The whole process starts with saliva. Saliva contains digestive enzymes that help break the chemical bonds holding foods together so they can be easily crushed and macerated by your teeth. These enzymes are pretty fast-acting; if you put a cracker or piece of toast on your tongue, you'll notice it quickly breaking down, even before you start to chew. Your tongue helps position the food in your mouth and moves it towards the back of your throat towards your oesophagus, the 10-inch connector between your mouth and your stomach. It's different from your windpipe, or trachea, which connects your mouth to your lungs. When you swallow, a little flap called the epiglottis covers the opening of the trachea to guard against choking. (If you've ever had food 'go down the wrong way', it's because your epiglottis didn't cover your trachea quickly enough.)

Once in the oesophagus, rhythmic automatic muscle contractions help push the food towards your stomach. There, acids further break down your meal, while your stomach muscles churn the whole mixture into what amounts to a nutrient-dense purée, which is then pushed into the 22-foot-long tunnel that is your small intestine. There, with the help of bile, a fat emulsifier produced by your gall bladder, and additional enzymes produced by your pancreas, your meal is absorbed through the walls of your intestine into your bloodstream in the form of individual nutrient building blocks – sugars, fatty acids and amino acids from carbohydrates, fats and proteins,

If I eat a pound of food, will I gain a pound in weight?

Three and a half pints of water weigh 4½lb but if you drink 3½ pints of water you won't put on 4lb of fat. You will, however, temporarily weigh 4lb more on the scales – that is, until your kidneys eliminate that water. That's because when you step on the scales, you are weighing anything that has weight to it – the water you just drank, the undigested food you ate a few hours ago, the waste from the food you ate yesterday that hasn't worked its way all the way through your GI tract yet, your muscle, skeleton, your body fat and the clothes you're wearing (if any).

Most of the weight fluctuations we see on the scales have to do with our fluid status, because that's the variable that changes the most from hour to hour and day to day. If you're retaining water, you could easily weigh 5lb more, and if you're dehydrated (maybe from being unwell), you could weigh 5lb less. Changes in actual body fat, however, happen much slower and are controlled solely by calories. It takes an excess of 3,500 calories (that means above and beyond the calories you burn) to create 1lb of body fat. If you ate 700 calories more than your body could burn in 1 day, you'd put on ⅕ of a pound. Do that for 5 days in a row starting on a Monday, and by the end of the working week, you've accumulated 1lb of fat. (By the way, this is nothing to sneeze at; it's only slightly less than 2 packets of butter!) So, while that number staring back at you seems to jump up and down like a yo-yo, you can see that it really takes several days in a row of overeating to even put on 1lb of actual body fat. The scale is much less fickle when it comes to fat than water!

respectively. Vitamins and minerals are also absorbed during the journey through the small intestine.

You may have noticed that I didn't mention dietary fibre. That's because you don't absorb fibre. Fibre fills you up, but doesn't add to your overall calorie intake. While fibre does contain as many calories as any other form of carbohydrate – about 4 per gram – your body isn't able to use them for energy. Instead, fibre just moves through your body nearly intact. Along the way, it binds to cholesterol, helping to shuttle it out of your system. A few studies have also found that fibre can prevent absorption of other calories you consume – up to 90 per day.

All the nutrients that do enter the bloodstream travel straight to the liver, which filters out wastes and decides where everything usable should go. Anything that isn't absorbed – fibre, waste by-products – travels down into the large intestine and finally through the colon and rectum. Before it leaves your body, small amounts of water and minerals are absorbed in a last-ditch effort to extract every last drop of importance out of that turkey sandwich.

Now that you're familiar with your GI tract, let's take a closer look at what's going on when you feel like a beach ball has taken up residence there.

Wind, Solids and Liquids: The Balloon Gang

THINK OF ONE of those very long, narrow balloons that you find at a child's birthday party, the ones that clowns twist into different shapes. That balloon represents your GI tract. Now picture the balloon filled with water, air or solid food. Each of these substances expands the balloon but does so in a different way.

■ AIR: When air enters the intestine – say, for example, from chewing gum, talking, drinking fizzy drinks or even smoking – it doesn't get absorbed into the bloodstream. Instead, it remains trapped until it can be eventually expelled via a belch or flatulence. Until then, it meanders through your GI tract, causing distension and discomfort.

DID YOU KNOW?

A calorie is a unit of energy needed to increase the temperature of 1 gram of water by 1°C. In everyday terms, it's energy that can have one of four origins and one of three destinations. There are four sources of calories: carbohydrates, protein, fat and alcohol. The first three types are essential to the body, but alcohol is not. When one of these types becomes available to the body, the cells will do one of three things with this energy. Basically, there is a priority system.

Fuel is the number one priority of every cell in the body. Just like cars need petrol, cells need fuel to perform their jobs (breathing, circulation, movement, etc.). Carbohydrate calories are the cells' preferred source of energy. The next priority is repair, healing and maintenance. Your body takes the energy from proteins and fats and uses them to patch up cells that are damaged or create new cells. Your muscles, bones, skin and immune system rely on protein and fat energy for this work. Finally, if all the cells are properly fuelled and repaired or replaced, your body takes the leftover or unneeded energy and stores it away in your fat cells.

When your body is in 'energy balance', it means the number of calories that showed up for work (the amount eaten) matched your needs perfectly. If you're in a positive energy balance, too many showed up and you end up storing some (i.e. weight gain); a negative energy balance means not enough calories are available. This can result in fatigue, feeling run-down and becoming ill or injured. The *Flat Belly Diet* is designed to keep you in balance – it provides enough energy in the form of carbohydrates, proteins and fats but not too much.

■ SOLID: It's generally just a matter of time before solid food gets broken down and absorbed or expelled. But until then, you're feeling like a beached whale.

■ LIQUID: Just like solid foods, liquid eventually gets absorbed, but sometimes we retain more fluid than our body really needs.

The Four Bad Boys of Bloat

THE FOUR-DAY ANTI-BLOAT Jumpstart has been created for the very specific purpose of eliminating wind, heavy solids and excess fluid so you will almost instantly feel and look lighter. Before we move on to the nitty-gritty details of the plan – what and when you'll eat – I want to explain four lifestyle factors that can also influence how prone you are to bloating or fluid retention.

1. STRESS: It triggers a complex sequence of hormonal fluctuations that raise blood pressure and divert blood to your extremities, where energy is most needed. This process allows you to run faster or lift more if necessary, but it also causes your digestive system to slow down significantly, which means you absorb nutrients more slowly (and sometimes miss some). As a result of the slowdown, your last meal may hang around in your intestine, causing bloat.

2. LACK OF FLUID: You've probably heard you need about eight glasses of water a day. Drinking water and even eating 'watery' foods like melon, green vegetables and other fruits and vegetables has enormous health benefits, including warding off fatigue, maintaining your body's proper fluid balance and guarding against water retention and constipation, which can cause bloating. Eight glasses is just a guideline; everyone's fluid needs vary according to activity level and body. Although all fluids (and water-packed foods) count towards your overall fluid intake, not all of these are permitted on the Four-Day Anti-Bloat Jumpstart.

3. LACK OF SLEEP: Too little sleep disrupts the intricate workings of your nervous system, which controls the rhythmic contractions of your GI tract and helps keep things humming along. It also affects your overall ability to manage and cope with stress. It's important to get at least 7 hours of sleep a night. If you have trouble sleeping, consult a sleep expert or visit the British Sleep Society's website at www.sleeping.org.uk

4. AIR TRAVEL: The average plane maintains cabin pressure equal to 5,000 to 8,000 feet above sea level in order to provide a comfortable atmosphere for the passengers. At that altitude, free air in the body cavities tends to expand by around 25 per cent.[1] Pressure changes also increase the production of gases in your GI tract. As the pressure in the cabin drops, the air in your intestines expands, causing bloating and discomfort. Cabin pressurization is also responsible for increased water retention because it impacts your body's natural fluid balance. Add in the dehydration caused by recirculated air and those bloat miles add up. Your best defence is to drink as much water as possible before and during your flight and to walk around as often as you can.

A Thinner, Lighter You in Four Days!

THE FOUR-DAY ANTI-BLOAT Jumpstart literally abolishes the foods, beverages and behaviours that cause your belly to paunch out. And – as a bonus – it provides guidelines for reducing the chances of ever feeling this way again. As you experience this phase, remember that you're taking the first step of your journey towards a healthier lifestyle. It's not just a smaller dress size. Here's what you're really gaining:

▓ An easy, safe, food-based solution for the body part you most want to change

▓ A more intense focus on your long-term health

▓ A reduced risk of heart disease, diabetes and cancer

▓ A comprehensive understanding of what constitutes a healthy meal

▓ A more thoughtful approach to meals that virtually eliminates emotional eating

Remember: This Four-Day Anti-Bloat Jumpstart is designed to do away with both bloating and water retention. Losing bloat is not the same as burning fat (we'll tackle that in the next chapter!), but it still creates a major change in your appearance and confidence level.

That's not to say you won't lose some serious weight! And you'll start right now. If you follow the instructions provided for the next 4 days, we estimate

(continued on page 76)

ARE YOU PRONE TO BELLY BLOAT?

DISCOVER HOW SUSCEPTIBLE YOU ARE TO BELLY BLOAT AND WATER RETEN-
TION BY TAKING THIS SIMPLE QUIZ. WHEN YOU'RE FINISHED, ADD UP YOUR
SCORE AND COMPARE IT TO THE RATINGS ON THE OPPOSITE PAGE.

QUESTION	A	B
Do you tend to eat too quickly? If **yes**, add 1 point for every speedy meal you eat per day (e.g. if you eat 4 times a day and they're all eaten at rapid speed, put a 4 in column A). If **no**, place a 1 in column B.		
Do you believe you are lactose intolerant? If **yes**, place a 1 in column A. If **no**, place a 1 in column B.		
Do you tend to talk a lot while you eat? If **yes**, place a 1 in column A. If **no**, place a 1 in column B.		
Do you add table salt to your food? If **yes**, add 1 point for every salt-sprinkled meal you eat per day (e.g. if you eat 4 times a day and you salt each meal, put a 4 in column A). If **no**, place a 1 in column B.		
Do you regularly binge on carbs? In other words, do you have episodes of eating more than you usually would of carb-rich foods at least once a week? If **yes**, add 1 point for every high-carb binge you can recall over the past week. If **no**, place a 1 in column B.		
Add 1 point to column A for each of the following foods you eat at least once a week: beans, lentils, nuts, cauliflower, broccoli, Brussels sprouts, cabbage, onions, peppers, raw citrus fruits. If you don't eat any of these foods at least once a week, add a 1 to column B.		
Do you chew gum, including sugar-free? If **yes**, add 1 point for every piece of gum you chew per week (e.g. if you chew 1 piece a day, put a 7 in column A). If **no**, place a 1 in column B.		
Do you use sugar substitutes? If **yes**, add 1 point for every packet you use per day (e.g. if you use 2 in your morning coffee, place a 2 in column A). If **no**, place a 1 in column B.		
Do you eat sugar-free sweets? If **yes**, add 1 point for every serving of sugar-free food you eat per week (e.g. if you suck sugar-free sweets in the afternoon at work all week, place a 5 in column A). If **no**, place a 1 in column B.		
Do you suffer from sleep apnoea? If **yes**, add 1 point. If **no**, place a 1 in column B.		
Do you eat fried foods? If **yes**, add 1 point for every serving of fried foods you eat per week (e.g. if you treat yourself to chips only once a week, place a 1 in column A). If **no**, place a 1 in column B.		

QUESTION	A	B
Do you drink fizzy drinks? If **yes**, add 1 point for every can or bottle you drink per week (e.g. if you drink 2 diet colas a day, place a 14 in column A). If **no**, place a 1 in column B.		
Do you drink coffee, tea or acidic juice (orange or tomato) daily? If **yes**, add 1 point for every glass or mug you drink per week (e.g. if you drink 2 cups of coffee a day, place a 14 in column A). If **no**, place a 1 in column B.		
Would you rate your everyday stress level as high? If **yes**, place a 1 in column A. If **no**, place a 1 in column B.		
Add up your score in each column:	*TOTAL* from column A:	*TOTAL* from column B:

FINAL TOTAL (Subtract B score from A score): _____

IF YOU SCORED:

A NEGATIVE NUMBER: Congratulations! Your bloating risk is relatively low. You're already avoiding a lot of the foods and bad habits that contribute to excessive bloating and water retention. But that doesn't mean the Four-Day Anti-Bloat Jumpstart won't help you. You may not lose significant measurements, but you will still *feel* lighter and healthier and be on a better path to long-term well-being.

0–5: NOT SO BAD. You probably experience come-and-go bloat. It's what I like to call bloat-flow – one day you're swollen; a few days later, you've deflated again. The good news is that you can tame your tummy without making too many changes to your lifestyle. You should get some immediate gratification on the Four-Day Anti-Bloat Jumpstart.

5–10: You may experience a little withdrawal from your usual habits, but you'll be handsomely rewarded – you should experience a noticeable difference after just 2 days on the Jumpstart.

10+: Congratulations again! If you're confused, don't be. I say congratulations because you are perfectly suited to seeing fantastic results on the Four-Day Anti-Bloat Jumpstart, so you're virtually primed for success on the *Flat Belly Diet* as a whole. The Jumpstart itself is really a cleansing – of foods, drinks and behaviours – that cause your body to unnecessarily hang on to fluid or produce excess wind and waste. It's not a detox but a cleaner, simpler way to eat than you may be used to. And because of that, you're likely to see some major belly shrinkage.

When Bloating Gets Bad

Bloating is a common condition, but in some cases, it can be a sign of a more serious health problem. It's time to see a doctor when:

- Your symptoms don't improve on the Four-Day Anti-Bloat Jumpstart.
- You're suffering from chronic constipation, diarrhoea, nausea or vomiting.
- You have persistent abdominal or rectal pain or heartburn.
- You've lost weight without trying.
- You have a fever you can't explain.
- There is blood in your urine.

that you can expect to lose as much as 7lb and up to 5¾ inches from your waist, hips, thighs, bust and arms combined. *No sweat necessary.* That's right – no exercise is needed. I didn't make these numbers up. They are actual amounts lost, all calculated by an expert who weighed and measured our test panellists. Rest assured: this plan has been proven to work on real women just like you.

Four Days – What to Avoid

■ THE SALT SHAKER, SALT-BASED SEASONINGS AND HIGHLY PROCESSED FOODS: Water is attracted to sodium, so when you take in higher than usual amounts of sodium, you'll temporarily retain more fluid – which contributes to a sluggish feeling, a puffy appearance and extra water weight. Cutting back on sodium and boosting your water intake will help bring your body back into balance. It'll also help reduce your risks of hypertension (high blood pressure) and osteoporosis. If you find your food lacks flavour without a few shakes of salt, use the recommended salt-free seasonings.

■ EXCESS CARBS: As a back-up energy source, your muscles store a type of carbohydrate called glycogen. Every gram of glycogen is stored with about 3 grams of water. But unless you're running a marathon tomorrow, you don't need all this stockpiled fuel. Decrease your intake of high-carbohydrate foods such as pasta, bananas, bagels and pretzels to temporarily train your body to access this stored fuel and burn it off. At the same time, you'll be getting rid of all that excess stored fluid.

■ BULKY RAW FOODS: A 60-gram (2-ounce) serving of cooked carrots delivers the same nutrition as 115 grams (4 ounces) raw, but it takes up less room in your GI tract. Eat only cooked vegetables, smaller portions of unsweetened dried fruit and canned fruits in natural juice. This will allow you to meet your nutrient needs without expanding your GI tract with extra volume.

■ GASSY FOODS: Certain foods simply create more wind in your GI tract. They include beans and pulses, cauliflower, broccoli, Brussels sprouts, cabbage, onions, peppers and citrus fruits.

■ CHEWING GUM: You probably don't realize this, but when you chew gum, you swallow air. All that air gets trapped in your GI tract and causes pressure, bloating and belly expansion.

■ SUGAR ALCOHOLS: These sugar substitutes, which go by the names xylitol or maltitol, are often found in products like low-calorie or low-carb biscuits, sweets and energy bars because they taste sweet. Like fibre, your GI tract can't absorb most of them. That's good for your calorie bottom line but not so good for your belly. Sugar alcohols cause wind, abdominal distention, bloating and diarrhoea. Avoid them.

■ FRIED FOODS: Fatty foods, especially the fried variety, are digested more slowly, causing you to feel heavy and bloated.

DID YOU KNOW ?

One way to take up less space in your stomach is to think what you put into it. For example, 170 grams (6 ounces) of grapes takes up four times as much space as 45 grams (1½ ounces) of unsweetened raisins.

■ SPICY FOODS: Foods seasoned with black pepper, nutmeg, cloves, chilli powder, hot sauces, onions, garlic, mustard, fresh chillies, barbecue sauce, horseradish, ketchup, tomato sauce or vinegar can all stimulate the release of stomach acid, which can cause irritation.

■ FIZZY DRINKS: Where do you think all those bubbles end up? They gang up in your belly!

■ ALCOHOL, COFFEE, TEA, HOT COCOA AND ACIDIC FRUIT JUICES: Each of these high-acid beverages can irritate your GI tract, causing swelling.

Four Days – What to Do

■ FOLLOW THE FOUR-DAY PLAN EXACTLY. This includes four smaller meals, one of which is a refreshing smoothie. This reduces the amount of food in your digestive system at any one time, cuts back on the release of stomach acids, and gets your body used to a four-meal-a-day schedule (which you'll be following on the rest of the *Flat Belly Diet*).

■ EAT FOUR MEALS A DAY. The Jumpstart includes fewer calories – about 1,200 daily – than you'll be eating on the *Flat Belly Diet*, which allows about 1,600 per day. Eating less for these 4 days reduces the amount of food in your GI tract at any one time, cuts back on the release of stomach acids and gets your body used to a four-meal-a-day schedule.

You'll notice a few staples, including sunflower seeds, flaxseed (linseed) oil, string cheese and carrots. There are three reasons you'll see these items appear repeatedly. First, we tried to limit the amount of food you have to buy to get started – and ensure you'll eat it before it goes bad. Second, we wanted to deliver a lot of nutritional and bloat-free value for your money. Finally, we chose foods that need no added salt or condiments to taste good, so you won't be tempted to reach for one of these potential bloat-promoters.

■ TAKE A QUICK 5-MINUTE AFTER-MEAL WALK. Moving your body helps release air that has been trapped in your GI tract, relieving pressure

SASS FROM SASS

'My Personal Flat Belly Tricks'

I am very prone to water retention. I'm drawn to salty foods more than sweet ones, and whenever I have an especially salty treat (cinema popcorn, anyone?), I get 'puffy' for at least a day after. So if I have an early morning TV appearance, I'm extra careful about what I eat the night before – you can bet there's no soy sauce involved! Some of us are genetically more prone to this phenomenon than others – nothing you can do about that. Here are some things to keep in mind about water retention, whether it's been a regular companion or occasional nuisance for you.

Remember, it's not fat! A friend once called me in a panic saying she'd put on nearly 4lb in one day. I asked if she'd eaten all her usual meals plus an extra 14,000 calories – because that, my friends, is what you'd need to eat to put on that much body fat in a day. She hadn't been bingeing, and I'm guessing you don't, either. So don't beat yourself up about that kind of weight gain. It's just water retention, and you'll lose it again.

Know your own body. Keeping a journal can help you track certain patterns. You might be more prone to water retention during a certain part of your menstrual cycle, and writing it down will show you when and for how long you tend to hang on to that extra fluid.

Plan ahead. If you're going to be in your swimming costume or you just want to look your leanest, avoid salty foods for at least several days beforehand. This is one kind of weight change you can control completely.   – *Cynthia*

and bloating. All it takes is a leisurely stroll down your street, around your office building or around the shops; a quick walk with your dog, a neighbour or your family after dinner – anything that gets you moving for just 5 minutes. You can walk for longer if you like, but at least 5 minutes are needed to help get things moving inside your belly.

■ DRINK ONE WHOLE SERVING OF CYNTHIA'S REFRESHING SIGNATURE SASSY WATER EVERY DAY. We call it Sassy because it's much perkier than plain old water, just like Cynthia herself! But the ingredients in here aren't just for flavour: the ginger also helps calm and soothe your GI tract. Even more important: the simple act of making this Sassy Water every day will serve as a reminder for these 4 days that life is a little bit different, that things are going to change. It will keep you focused on the flat-belly task ahead. In addition, you may drink 100 per cent pure herbal teas such as camomile or peppermint.

SASSY WATER

2 litres (3½ pints) water
1 teaspoon freshly grated ginger
1 medium cucumber, peeled and thinly sliced
1 medium lemon, thinly sliced
12 mint leaves

Combine all ingredients in a large jug, chill in the refrigerator and let the flavours blend overnight.

■ EAT SLOWLY. Often, when you eat quickly, you take in large gulps of air without realizing it. All that excess air gets trapped in your digestive system and causes bloating (think of a balloon stretched to capacity). Taking your time will help prevent the expansion. It will also keep you calm, and allow you to connect with the concept of mealtime as a moment to stop, rest and reflect. Too often, we hurry through meals, always trying to get to the next block of time on our to-do schedule. Let's put an end to this for these 4 days, and beyond, and remember the joy that comes from respecting mealtimes.

■ WORK YOUR MIND. The first days of a diet are never easy, and these 4 days are no exception. I'm asking you to change how you eat and to give up some of the foods you're used to eating or drinking – and perhaps imagine you can't live without. Of course, it's going to be worth it in the end – it does work and you will see your belly shrink. But until you see that paunch disappear, you'll need a mental tune-up. That's where my Mind Tricks come in.

Your Four-Day Shopping List

PRODUCE
- ❏ 460g (16½oz) cherry tomatoes
- ❏ 230g (8oz) fresh or frozen green beans
- ❏ 2 large red potatoes
- ❏ 230g (8oz) baby carrots
- ❏ 115g (4oz) button mushrooms
- ❏ 1 large yellow squash or courgette
- ❏ 4 medium cucumbers
- ❏ 4 medium lemons

DAIRY
- ❏ 2 litres (3½ pints) skimmed milk
- ❏ 1 packet light string cheese

FRUIT
- ❏ 115g (4oz) blueberries, fresh or frozen (no added sugar)
- ❏ 115g (4oz) peaches, frozen or tinned in their own juices (no added sugar)
- ❏ 115g (4oz) pears, frozen or tinned in their own juices (no added sugar)
- ❏ 115g (4oz) strawberries, fresh, frozen or tinned in their own juices (no added sugar)

DRY GOODS
- ❏ 375g (13oz) box unsweetened cornflakes
- ❏ 375g (13oz) box unsweetened puffed rice cereal
- ❏ 1 packet (27g/1oz) Oats So Simple®, original variety
- ❏ 230g (8oz) box brown (wholegrain) rice

- ❏ 230g (8oz) tin pineapple chunks in juice (no added sugar)
- ❏ 1 packet (approx 115g/4oz) roasted or raw unsalted sunflower seeds
- ❏ 240ml (8fl oz) bottle cold-pressed organic flaxseed (linseed) oil
- ❏ 240ml (8fl oz) bottle olive oil
- ❏ small bag unsweetened raisins
- ❏ small bag prunes

HERBS AND SPICES
- ❏ 1–2 pieces fresh ginger root
- ❏ 2 bunches fresh mint

MEAT/SEAFOOD
- ❏ 3 packets organic turkey slices
- ❏ 115g (4oz) cod or pollack
- ❏ 170g (6oz) boneless skinless chicken breast
- ❏ 90g (3oz) turkey breast fillet
- ❏ 90g (3oz) tinned tuna in water

ANY OF THESE APPROVED SALT-FREE SEASONINGS
- ❏ Fresh or dried: basil, bay leaf, cinnamon, curry powder, dill, ginger, lemon or lime juice, marjoram, mint, oregano, paprika, pepper, rosemary, sage, tarragon or thyme
- ❏ Aged balsamic vinegar

Mind Tricks are a way of giving a meal importance – making it a special, you-focused moment. They'll help you stay watchful about what you're eating and why. As you embark on the 4 days' worth of Mind Tricks – 16 in all, one at every meal – you'll surely find some that are so appealing that you'll want to repeat them again and again. In fact, you should repeat your favourites until they become a ritual. I'm all for doing whatever it takes to make you feel special.

Track Your Progress

STUDIES HAVE REGULARLY shown that keeping a log of what you eat and how you feel while you're eating helps you stay on track with new lifestyle choices. There is now increasing evidence to support the concept that keeping a journal has a positive impact on physical well-being. University of Texas at Austin researcher Dr James Pennebaker has scientifically shown that keeping a journal regularly strengthens immune cells called T-lymphocytes.[2] Other research indicates that keeping a journal may help decrease the symptoms of asthma and rheumatoid arthritis. Pennebaker believes that writing about stressful events helps you come to terms with them, thus reducing the impact of these stressors on your physical health.

SASS FROM SASS

'Measure your food'

Always measure foods – especially those that pack a lot of calories in small amounts, including oil, nuts, seeds, peanut butter, avocado, pasta, rice and porridge oats. Measuring will help ensure that this carefully calculated plan gives you the results you're looking for. Without measuring, it's very easy to miscalculate and rack up hundreds of extra calories. I've certainly seen this in my practice as a registered dietitian.   – *Cynthia*

But in addition to all those things, keeping a journal is a simple way to feel as if you're making significant progress. When I was training for a marathon, one of the biggest motivators in getting me into my running shoes and out of the door every morning was my running log. All I wanted to do was fill in the log, and I would get engrossed in watching the mileage accumulate week after week. Similarly, a journal will inspire you to focus on and achieve your weight loss goals.

For the Four-Day Anti-Bloat Jumpstart, your journal is incorporated into your meal plan. Later, when you complete the Jumpstart and begin the *Flat Belly Diet*, I'll ask you to spend a bit more time filling in your journal about specific issues that you may have about food and your body confidence. For now, take these 4 days to get used to the format of the food journal – and start building the habit of sitting down and recording everything you've put into your mouth that day.

A few rules of keeping a journal:

1. Forget spelling and punctuation.
2. Write quickly to ward off your inner critic.
3. Speak from your heart.

Day Four and Beyond

AS YOU REACH the final day of your Anti-Bloat Jumpstart, I know what you'll be feeling. You'll feel lighter, stronger, more confident and more self-centred (in a good way) than you've ever felt before. That's exactly the right mindset for forging ahead and beginning the next phase of the *Flat Belly Diet:* the 28-day programme that will give you the tools to manage your health and maintain your desired goal weight for the rest of your life.

THE FOUR-DAY ANTI-BLOAT MENU, DAY 1

DATE:

BREAKFAST

- ❏ 30g (1oz) unsweetened cornflakes
- ❏ 240ml (8fl oz) skimmed milk
- ❏ 115g (4oz) tinned pears in natural juice (no added sugar)
- ❏ 30g (1oz) roasted or raw unsalted sunflower seeds
- ❏ Glass of Sassy Water

MIND TRICK: Say hello, sunshine! Enjoy breakfast near a sunny window. Morning sunlight has been shown to be a mood booster and will set your body's master clock for maximum all-day energy.

LUNCH

- ❏ 115g (4oz) organic turkey slices, rolled up
- ❏ 1 light string cheese
- ❏ 230g (8oz) fresh cherry tomatoes
- ❏ Glass of Sassy Water

MIND TRICK: Put some colour in your day. Before sitting down, arrange a few cut flowers in a vase and place it on the table. You're working hard on this diet. You deserve something special for your efforts.

SNACK

- ❏ Blueberry Smoothie: Blend 240ml (8fl oz) skimmed milk and 115g (4oz) fresh or frozen unsweetened blueberries in blender for 1 minute. Transfer to glass and stir in 1tbsp cold-pressed organic flaxseed (linseed) oil, or serve with 1tbsp sunflower or pumpkin seeds.

MIND TRICK: Take a virtual holiday. Put on some reggae music while you're preparing your meal and transport yourself to a beach with lapping water and coconut palms. For good measure rub a little suntan oil on your face and inhale deeply. It's snowing outside? No. You're in the Caribbean.

DINNER

- ❏ 115g (4oz) cooked green beans
- ❏ 115g (4oz) grilled cod or pollack
- ❏ 60g (2oz) roast potatoes drizzled with 1tsp olive oil
- ❏ Glass of Sassy Water

MIND TRICK: Resize your settings. Set your table with smaller plates and bowls. It'll make you feel like you have more food than you actually do.

JOURNAL, DAY 1

DATE:

BREAKFAST	
MOOD:	THOUGHTS/CHALLENGES:

HUNGER BEFORE: -5 -3 0 3 5 7 | HUNGER AFTER: -5 -3 0 3 5 7

LUNCH	
MOOD:	THOUGHTS/CHALLENGES:

HUNGER BEFORE: -5 -3 0 3 5 7 | HUNGER AFTER: -5 -3 0 3 5 7

SNACK	
MOOD:	THOUGHTS/CHALLENGES:

HUNGER BEFORE: -5 -3 0 3 5 7 | HUNGER AFTER: -5 -3 0 3 5 7

DINNER	
MOOD:	THOUGHTS/CHALLENGES:

HUNGER BEFORE: -5 -3 0 3 5 7 | HUNGER AFTER: -5 -3 0 3 5 7

Hunger Rating

-5 = STARVING. You want to devour the first thing you see and have a hard time slowing down.

-3 = OVERLY HUNGRY AND IRRITABLE. You feel like you waited too long to eat.

0 = MILD TO MODER-ATE HUNGER. You may have physical symptoms of hunger, like a growling tummy and that 'I need to eat soon' feeling, but you aren't starving or experiencing any unpleasant symptoms such as a headache or shaking.

3 = HUNGER- BUT NOT CRAVING-FREE. You're full, but you don't feel quite satisfied; your thoughts are still focused on food.

5 = JUST RIGHT. Your hunger is gone, and you feel satisfied. Your mind is off food, and you're ready to take on the next task. You feel energized.

7 = A LITTLE TOO MUCH. You think you overdid it. Your tummy feels stretched and uncomfortable. You feel kind of sluggish.

THE FOUR-DAY ANTI-BLOAT MENU, DAY 2

DATE:

BREAKFAST

- ❑ 30g (1oz) unsweetened puffed rice cereal
- ❑ 240ml (8fl oz) skimmed milk
- ❑ 30g (1oz) roasted or raw unsalted sunflower seeds
- ❑ 115g (4oz) tinned pineapple chunks in natural juice
- ❑ Glass of Sassy Water

MIND TRICK: Find a one-meal-only mantra. Pick a calming word or phrase, such as 'I'm doing this diet for me.' Repeat it after every bite.

LUNCH

- ❑ 90g (3oz) tinned tuna in water
- ❑ 115g (4oz) steamed baby carrots
- ❑ 1 light string cheese
- ❑ Glass of Sassy Water

MIND TRICK: Convert a friend. Invite a pal to have lunch with you today and explain your meal. Try to remember as many principles of the Jumpstart as possible. This will help you remember why you're doing this, even though it's such a departure from your normal routine.

SNACK

- ❑ Pineapple Smoothie: Blend 240ml (8fl oz) skimmed milk, 115g (4oz) tinned pineapple chunks in juice, and a handful of ice in blender for 1 minute. Transfer to glass and stir in 1tbsp cold-pressed organic flaxseed (linseed) oil, or serve with 1 tbsp sunflower or pumpkin seeds.

MIND TRICK: Hang up some inspiration. Keep, say, your 'skinny jeans' on a hanger in full view, so you pass them every day. They'll serve as a reminder of your ultimate weight loss goal. They *will* fit you again.

DINNER

- ❑ 115g (4oz) fresh button mushrooms sautéed with 1tsp olive oil
- ❑ 90g (3oz) grilled chicken breast
- ❑ 110g (3½oz) cooked brown rice
- ❑ Glass of Sassy Water

MIND TRICK: Sing while you prepare dinner. According to German researchers, you can enjoy up to a 240 per cent immunity boost as well as an increase of anti-stress hormones simply by singing.

JOURNAL, DAY 2

DATE: ....

BREAKFAST	
MOOD:	THOUGHTS/CHALLENGES:

HUNGER BEFORE: -5 -3 0 3 5 7 | HUNGER AFTER: -5 -3 0 3 5 7

LUNCH	
MOOD:	THOUGHTS/CHALLENGES:

HUNGER BEFORE: -5 -3 0 3 5 7 | HUNGER AFTER: -5 -3 0 3 5 7

SNACK	
MOOD:	THOUGHTS/CHALLENGES:

HUNGER BEFORE: -5 -3 0 3 5 7 | HUNGER AFTER: -5 -3 0 3 5 7

DINNER	
MOOD:	THOUGHTS/CHALLENGES:

HUNGER BEFORE: -5 -3 0 3 5 7 | HUNGER AFTER: -5 -3 0 3 5 7

Hunger Rating

–5 = STARVING. You want to devour the first thing you see and have a hard time slowing down.

–3 = OVERLY HUNGRY AND IRRITABLE. You feel like you waited too long to eat.

0 = MILD TO MODERATE HUNGER. You may have physical symptoms of hunger, like a growling tummy and that 'I need to eat soon' feeling, but you aren't starving or experiencing any unpleasant symptoms such as a headache or shaking.

3 = HUNGER- BUT NOT CRAVING-FREE. You're full, but you don't feel quite satisfied; your thoughts are still focused on food.

5 = JUST RIGHT. Your hunger is gone, and you feel satisfied. Your mind is off food, and you're ready to take on the next task. You feel energized.

7 = A LITTLE TOO MUCH. You think you overdid it. Your tummy feels stretched and uncomfortable. You feel kind of sluggish.

THE FOUR-DAY ANTI-BLOAT MENU, DAY 3

DATE:

BREAKFAST

- ❏ 30g (1oz) unsweetened cornflakes
- ❏ 240ml (8fl oz) skimmed milk
- ❏ 30g (1oz) roasted or raw unsalted sunflower seeds
- ❏ 2tbsp raisins
- ❏ Glass of Sassy Water

MIND TRICK: Focus on your moment. This morning, eat your breakfast with no distraction – no radio, no morning show, no newspaper. Focus on the flavour of each bite.

LUNCH

- ❏ 115g (4oz) organic turkey slices, rolled up
- ❏ 1 light string cheese
- ❏ 230g (8oz) cherry tomatoes
- ❏ Glass of Sassy Water

MIND TRICK: Bring in some bling. Serve your Sassy Water in the finest crystal glass you own. Make this your Flat Belly glass, and use it at every meal.

SNACK

- ❏ Peach Smoothie: Blend 240ml (8fl oz) skimmed milk and 115g (4oz) frozen or tinned, unsweetened peaches in blender for 1 minute. Transfer to glass and stir in 1tbsp cold-pressed organic flaxseed (linseed) oil, or serve with 1tbsp sunflower or pumpkin seeds.

MIND TRICK: Give thanks. Take a moment of gratitude for the food you are eating, the body you are nurturing and the life you're enhancing. No need to get religious – it's perfectly OK to thank the peach farmer and your parents!

DINNER

- ❏ 115g (4oz) cooked green beans
- ❏ 90g (3oz) grilled or baked turkey breast cutlet
- ❏ 60g (2oz) roast potatoes drizzled with 1tsp olive oil
- ❏ Glass of Sassy Water

MIND TRICK: Think about yourself. Remember the list you compiled in Chapter 4, the one listing all the important people in your life? As you eat this meal, reflect on all you're doing to care for your body and your spirit.

JOURNAL, DAY 3

DATE:

BREAKFAST	
MOOD:	THOUGHTS/CHALLENGES:

HUNGER BEFORE: -5 -3 0 3 5 7 | HUNGER AFTER: -5 -3 0 3 5 7

LUNCH	
MOOD:	THOUGHTS/CHALLENGES:

HUNGER BEFORE: -5 -3 0 3 5 7 | HUNGER AFTER: -5 -3 0 3 5 7

SNACK	
MOOD:	THOUGHTS/CHALLENGES:

HUNGER BEFORE: -5 -3 0 3 5 7 | HUNGER AFTER: -5 -3 0 3 5 7

DINNER	
MOOD:	THOUGHTS/CHALLENGES:

HUNGER BEFORE: -5 -3 0 3 5 7 | HUNGER AFTER: -5 -3 0 3 5 7

Hunger Rating

–5 = STARVING. You want to devour the first thing you see and have a hard time slowing down.

–3 = OVERLY HUNGRY AND IRRITABLE. You feel like you waited too long to eat.

0 = MILD TO MODER-ATE HUNGER. You may have physical symptoms of hunger, like a growling tummy and that 'I need to eat soon' feeling, but you aren't starving or experiencing any unpleasant symptoms such as a headache or shaking.

3 = HUNGER- BUT NOT CRAVING-FREE. You're full, but you don't feel quite satisfied; your thoughts are still focused on food.

5 = JUST RIGHT. Your hunger is gone, and you feel satisfied. Your mind is off food, and you're ready to take on the next task. You feel energized.

7 = A LITTLE TOO MUCH. You think you overdid it. Your tummy feels stretched and uncomfortable. You feel kind of sluggish.

THE FOUR-DAY ANTI-BLOAT MENU, DAY 4

DATE:

<table>
<tr><td colspan="2">BREAKFAST</td></tr>
<tr>
<td>

❑ 1 packet Oats So Simple®, original variety

❑ 240ml (8fl oz) skimmed milk

❑ 30g (1oz) roasted or raw unsalted sunflower seeds

❑ 2 prunes

❑ Glass of Sassy Water

</td>
<td>

MIND TRICK: Have a laugh. A 4-year-old laughs around 400 times a day; an adult, around 15. Today, even if you're alone when you sit down to your meal, laugh at your bowl of Oats So Simple, howl at your glass of Sassy Water.

</td>
</tr>
</table>

<table>
<tr><td colspan="2">LUNCH</td></tr>
<tr>
<td>

❑ 115g (4oz) organic turkey slices, rolled up

❑ 115g (4oz) steamed baby carrots

❑ 1 light string cheese

❑ Glass of Sassy Water

</td>
<td>

MIND TRICK: Arrange your plate. Take a few minutes to prepare today's lunch with the flair of a gourmet chef. Wrap the turkey slices around the cheese and carrots, then slice on the bias and arrange. Garnish with a few sprigs of fresh herbs.

</td>
</tr>
</table>

<table>
<tr><td colspan="2">SNACK</td></tr>
<tr>
<td>

❑ Strawberry Smoothie: Blend 240ml (8fl oz) skimmed milk and 115g (4oz) fresh or frozen, unsweetened strawberries in blender for 1 minute. Transfer to glass and stir in 1tbsp cold-pressed organic flaxseed (linseed) oil, or serve with 1tbsp sunflower or pumpkin seeds.

</td>
<td>

MIND TRICK: Before you sit down to eat, close your eyes and say something kind and reassuring about your body. Mention how much you love your arms or how people tell you you have great eyes or a fantastic smile.

</td>
</tr>
</table>

<table>
<tr><td colspan="2">DINNER</td></tr>
<tr>
<td>

❑ 115g (4oz) yellow squash or courgettes sautéed with 1tsp olive oil

❑ 90g (3oz) grilled chicken breast

❑ 110g (3½oz) cooked brown rice

❑ Glass of Sassy Water

</td>
<td>

MIND TRICK: Serve today's dinner on your best china. Set a proper place setting with the good silver and the linen napkins.

</td>
</tr>
</table>

JOURNAL, DAY 4

DATE:

BREAKFAST	
MOOD:	THOUGHTS/CHALLENGES:

HUNGER BEFORE: -5 -3 0 3 5 7 | HUNGER AFTER: -5 -3 0 3 5 7

LUNCH	
MOOD:	THOUGHTS/CHALLENGES:

HUNGER BEFORE: -5 -3 0 3 5 7 | HUNGER AFTER: -5 -3 0 3 5 7

SNACK	
MOOD:	THOUGHTS/CHALLENGES:

HUNGER BEFORE: -5 -3 0 3 5 7 | HUNGER AFTER: -5 -3 0 3 5 7

DINNER	
MOOD:	THOUGHTS/CHALLENGES:

HUNGER BEFORE: -5 -3 0 3 5 7 | HUNGER AFTER: -5 -3 0 3 5 7

Hunger Rating

-5 = STARVING. You want to devour the first thing you see and have a hard time slowing down.

-3 = OVERLY HUNGRY AND IRRITABLE. You feel like you waited too long to eat.

0 = MILD TO MODERATE HUNGER. You may have physical symptoms of hunger, like a growling tummy and that 'I need to eat soon' feeling, but you aren't starving or experiencing any unpleasant symptoms such as a headache or shaking.

3 = HUNGER- BUT NOT CRAVING-FREE. You're full, but you don't feel quite satisfied; your thoughts are still focused on food.

5 = JUST RIGHT. Your hunger is gone, and you feel satisfied. Your mind is off food, and you're ready to take on the next task. You feel energized.

7 = A LITTLE TOO MUCH. You think you overdid it. Your tummy feels stretched and uncomfortable. You feel kind of sluggish.

Four-Day Anti-Bloat Jumpstart Success

Congratulations! You've completed the first phase of the Flat Belly Diet. Take a little time now to weigh and measure yourself, and see how much you've lost in just these four days!

Before you plunge into the main phase of the Flat Belly Diet, reflect on your experience with the Four-Day Anti-Bloat Jumpstart. What were the hardest things for you to cope with? What turned out to be not as bad as you had feared? When did hunger rear its head (or did it)? Which mind tricks helped the most? These lessons will help set the stage for your success during the next 28 days.

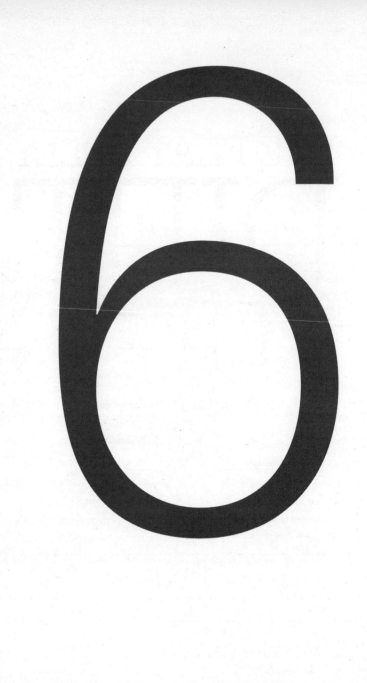

THE FLAT BELLY
DIET
RULES

WOW. Isn't it amazing how dramatically you can change the way you think and feel in only 4 short days? You've just completed a major milestone on the *Flat Belly Diet* – you've mastered the elusive art of banishing bloat from your life for ever. And, if you completed each Mind Trick, you've accumulated lots of little useful strategies you can employ anywhere, any time, to boost your confidence and stay motivated. But now that you've seen how a flatter belly looks and felt the renewed confidence that comes from experiencing such fast results, you're ready to move on to the next – and most life-changing – phase of the *Flat Belly Diet:* you're ready to lose belly fat.

For just about everyone who's ever tried to lose weight, the word *diet* means long lists of forbidden foods, non-stop hunger, willpower struggles and, eventually, a return to 'normal' eating once you've met your goal. For Cynthia and me, *diet* has an altogether different meaning, one that's inspired by the US National Institutes of Health, which simply defines diet as 'what a person eats and drinks; a type of eating plan'. The *Flat Belly Diet* is a way of eating, one that allows you to get to, and then stay at, your ideal weight, while optimizing your health and energy and slashing your odds of getting nearly every chronic disease.

Our plan, as you know, makes a specific promise: less belly fat. And less belly fat will, in turn, reduce your risk of disease. But even after we'd found the research supporting the notion that a particular food group – those beloved MUFAs – could accomplish that, and even after Cynthia worked out the calorie counts and made sure that the nutrient requirements of the average woman could be met, we still had a bit of work to do. I knew that the *Flat Belly Diet* was going to have to compete with a whole shelf (or many shelves) full of popular plans, every one of them promising significant weight loss. I knew that to stand out on that shelf, it had to offer something – or many things – that other diets don't have.

Step one was asking women what they loved and hated about traditional weight-loss diets. I quickly found that one woman's dietary nightmare is another's dream, which is probably why there's a diet book for every woman out there these days. Books exist for people with certain blood types, people who hate carbs, people with fat phobias, people who like, um, cabbage soup – whoever those unique and adventurous individuals might be. But I talked to Cynthia and learned a few universal truths about diets that actually work for the vast majority of people.

- They offer sound advice and deliver on their promises. (Check. I would offer you nothing less.)
- They offer a plan that women can return to again and again, whenever their favourite jeans feel a little too snug. (Check. The Four-Day Anti-

Bloat Jumpstart is an effective, safe solution you can turn to whenever
you need an instant svelting.)

■ They are easy to live with. (Check . . . ?)

Ahhh, that was the rub: how could we devise a plan that worked for every-
body all the time? I thought about this for a long time and worried that it
wasn't possible simply because there are as many definitions of 'perfect' as
there are readers of this book. Cynthia assured me, however, that it *was* possible! Her years of counselling dieters – and her rigorous planning for the
Flat Belly Diet – are the backbone of this lifestyle. It was possible because
the *Flat Belly Diet* offers:

■ FOCUS ON HEALTH AND ENERGY. Anyone can lose weight on a
1,200-calorie diet. But here's what you'll also lose: muscle, bone density, zest
for living, sanity and, if you follow a diet like that for too long, your sense of
humour. (I've seen it happen!) Featuring satisfying, wholesome foods and a
1,600-calorie-a-day guideline, the *Flat Belly Diet* is as healthy as they come.

■ FLAVOUR. It's food, after all! We consider no diet 'complete' or
'healthy' unless it's filled with delicious foods and meals any palate can
enjoy. This plan offers as much taste as nutrition.

■ REALITY. We wouldn't ask anyone to do something that we weren't
willing – or able – to do ourselves.

■ FLEXIBILITY. If you're pressed for time, we want you to be able to
assemble meals quickly, with little or no cooking. If, on the other hand,

you want to cook for your family or friends, we wanted to make that easy without endangering your goal. And finally, if you don't like a suggested meal, you should be able to swap it for something you *do* want to eat. The *Flat Belly Diet* is about as flexible as it gets.

Three Rules to Eat By

OVER THE NEXT 28 days – and beyond – you are going to eat very well. How does Spicy Prawns with Chilli Bean Glaze sound? Chicago-Style Hot Dog, anyone? How about a Red Fruit Crumble? They're just a few of the anti-'diet' dishes you'll be eating. And it won't be a lot of work. We've developed two different ways to follow the *Flat Belly Diet:* the first, in Chapter 7, is perfect if you're too busy to even think about cooking dinner. It's also a great way to familiarize yourself with this new way of eating, because it lays everything out for you. You don't have to think about portion size because everything is pre-portioned. Chapter 8 is loaded with MUFA-packed recipes and meal additions that will allow you to follow the *Flat Belly Diet* when convenience foods may not be an option – family dinner night, for example, or when you're entertaining. Both plans adhere to three very important *Flat Belly Diet* rules that you must follow if you expect to reap the health and weight-loss rewards on this plan. They are:

- ■ Rule #1: Stick to 400 calories per meal.

- ■ Rule #2: Never go more than 4 hours without eating.

- ■ Rule #3: Eat a MUFA at every meal.

RULE #1: STICK TO 400 CALORIES PER MEAL

YOU'VE PROBABLY NOTICED from looking at the list of MUFAs on page 37 that they're not exactly low-cal choices. They're all foods – nuts, oils, chocolate – that you're usually told to avoid when you're trying to lose weight. But because these MUFAs are so essential to losing belly fat, calorie control in what surrounds them takes on extra importance. All the meals in the *Flat Belly Diet* provide a MUFA *and* total about 400 calories. An added bonus of this controlled-calorie plan is that you can substitute one whole meal for another. You can eat breakfast for dinner or lunch for breakfast. If you like, you can even eat four breakfast meals in one day. That's part of the ease of this plan. I don't expect that you'll love every single meal. But on the other hand, if you find a few you absolutely adore, it's perfectly OK to enjoy them to your heart's content.

This diet is 1,600 calories per day because that's how much it takes for a woman of average height, frame size and activity level to get to and stay at her ideal body weight. So 1,600 calories is not a starvation plan – it's enough to keep up your energy, support your immune system and maintain your precious calorie-burning muscle. That means you won't feel run-down, irritable, moody or hungry. But you also won't be eating enough calories to hang on to your belly.

RULE #2: NEVER GO MORE THAN
4 HOURS WITHOUT EATING

I DON'T HAVE to tell you that a diet won't work if it makes you feel hungry or tired. That's why, on the *Flat Belly Diet*, you're *required* to eat every 4 hours. Waiting too long to eat can cause you to become so hungry (and irritable) that it's hard to even think clearly. That means you won't have the energy or patience to think through the healthiest meal choice, let alone prepare one. You'll probably want to tear into the first thing you see (bag of crisps, handfuls of dry cereal straight from the box, biscuits and so on), and you'll probably have a hard time slowing down while you eat and not reaching for seconds.

Snacks are especially important, but when you eat them is entirely up to you. I like to have a snack in the evening while I'm reading manuscripts, but some of the editors I work with need a small meal in the afternoon to keep them going until dinnertime. Your snack time is entirely personal and entirely essential. To help you include your snack every day, Cynthia has created a variety of Snack Packs that you can prepare in advance and take with you each morning. They're portable and MUFA-loaded. Use the Snack Pack as a floating meal.

RULE #3: EAT A MUFA AT EVERY MEAL

'A MUFA AT every meal' has almost become a mantra for me. As you know, 'MUFA' (MOO-fah) stands for 'monounsaturated fatty acid', a type of heart-healthy, disease-fighting, 'good' fat found in foods like almonds, peanut butter, olive oil, avocados, even chocolate. MUFAs are an *un*saturated fat and have the exact opposite effect of the unhealthy saturated and trans fats you've heard about in the news.

But there's more! MUFAs are delicious in and of themselves. Who doesn't love drizzling olive oil over a salad or grabbing a handful of chocolate chips? You'll find the MUFA-rich foods incorporated into the meal plans and Snack Packs. You can substitute one MUFA for another as long as the calorie counts are nearly equivalent. For example, you can exchange almond butter (200 calories) for dark chocolate chips (210). For precise MUFA serving amounts per meal, consult the chart on the opposite page. Better still, copy this chart and stick it on the inside door of your kitchen cupboard. To get better acquainted with the five MUFA groups and learn how to buy, store and prepare them, turn to page 103.

YOUR MUFA SERVING CHART

FOOD	SERVING	CALORIES
SOYA BEANS (EDAMAME), SHELLED AND BOILED	190g (6½oz)	244
DARK CHOCOLATE CHIPS	45g (1½oz)	210
ALMOND BUTTER	2tbsp	200
CASHEW BUTTER	2tbsp	190
SUNFLOWER SEED BUTTER	2tbsp	190
NATURAL PEANUT BUTTER, CRUNCHY	2tbsp	188
NATURAL PEANUT BUTTER, SMOOTH	2tbsp	188
TAHINI (SESAME SEED PASTE)	2tbsp	178
PUMPKIN SEEDS	2tbsp	148
RAPESEED (CANOLA) OIL	1tbsp	124
FLAXSEED (LINSEED) OIL (COLD-PRESSED ORGANIC)	1tbsp	120
MACADAMIA NUTS	2tbsp	120
SAFFLOWER OIL (HIGH OLEIC)	1tbsp	120
SESAME OIL	1tbsp	120
SUNFLOWER OIL (HIGH OLEIC)	1tbsp	120
WALNUT OIL	1tbsp	120
OLIVE OIL	1tbsp	119
PEANUT (GROUNDNUT) OIL	1tbsp	119
PINE NUTS	2tbsp	113
BRAZIL NUTS	2tbsp	110
HAZELNUTS	2tbsp	110
PEANUTS	2tbsp	110
ALMONDS	2tbsp	109
CASHEWS	2tbsp	100
AVOCADO (HASS)	60g (2oz)	96
PECANS	2 tbsp	90
SUNFLOWER SEEDS	2 tbsp	90
BLACK OLIVE TAPENADE	2 tbsp	88
PISTACHIOS	2 tbsp	88
WALNUTS	2 tbsp	82
PESTO SAUCE	1 tbsp	80
AVOCADO, GREEN (FLORIDA)	60g (2oz)	69
GREEN OLIVE TAPENADE	2 tbsp	54
GREEN OR BLACK OLIVES	10 large	50

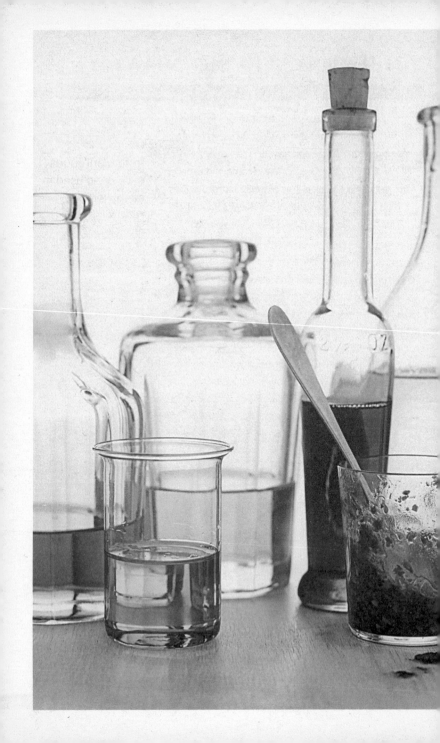

1. Oils

ANOINT YOUR MEALS with the most versatile MUFAs in the kitchen. Choose your oil based on use – cooking or drizzling – and flavour – strong or mild. HOW TO BUY AND USE: We recommend expeller pressed oils, a chemical-free extraction process. This natural method allows the oil to retain its natural colour, aroma and nutrients. Cold-pressed oil is expeller pressed in a heat-controlled environment to keep temperatures below 49°C (120°F). This is important for delicate oils like flaxseed (linseed). HOW TO STORE: Choose a container that holds only what you'll use within 2 months. As each container empties, it fills with oxygen, which causes the oil to oxidize, or deteriorate. This eventually creates a stale or bitter taste (like wet cardboard) and contributes to a breakdown of vitamin E and those precious MUFAs. Opt for dark glass jars or tins (rather than clear plastic bottles) to protect the oil from light, another source of flavour-sapping oxidation. You can store opened bottles of olive, rapeseed (canola) and peanut (groundnut) oils in a dark, cool place, such as the back of your larder, but flaxseed (linseed) oil should always be kept in the refrigerator because it breaks down more quickly at warmer temperatures.

HISTORY

Oils extracted from plant foods have been used in nearly every culture around the globe since ancient times. A 4,000-year-old kitchen unearthed by an archaeologist in Indiana revealed that large slabs of rock had been used to crush nuts, then extract the oil.

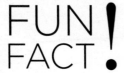

FUN FACT !

SAFFLOWER OIL LABELLED 'HIGH-OLEIC' CONTAINS THE MOST BENEFICIAL MUFAS, FOLLOWED BY OLIVE OIL AND THEN RAPESEED (CANOLA) OIL.

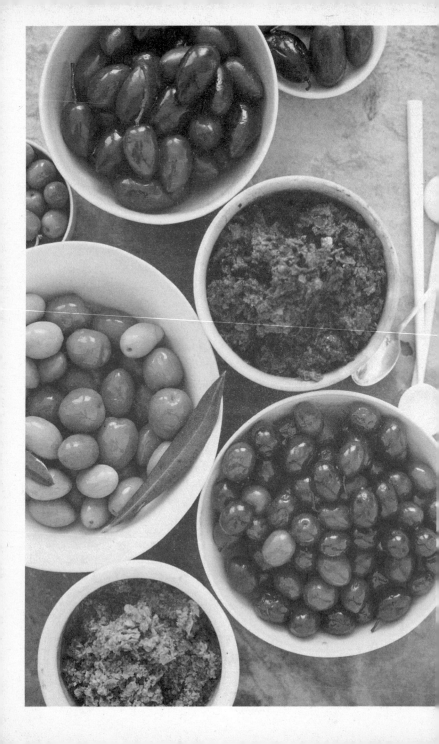

2. Olives

THERE'S AN OLIVE out there just for you. Choose your colour (black or green) and pick your flavour (salty, sweet or spicy). When you're all olived out, switch to tapenade, a deliciously pungent spread made from the crushed fruit.

HOW TO BUY AND USE: Choose your olives from deli counters; they are sometimes pasteurized and cured in either oil, salt or brine, and flavoured with herbs or hot chillies. Olives can be purchased in jars and tins, as well as in bulk.

HOW TO STORE: Olives should be stored in the refrigerator after opening, either in the jar or an airtight container. If you bought your olives in tins, transfer any leftovers into another airtight container before storing in the fridge.

HISTORY

Native to coastal regions of the Mediterranean, Asia and areas of Africa, olives have been cultivated since 6000 BC and are one of the oldest known foods. These gems were distributed around the world by Spanish and Portuguese explorers during the 15th and 16th centuries. Today, most commercial olives are grown in Spain, Italy, Greece and Turkey.

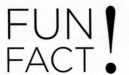

FUN FACT !

TRADITIONAL CHINESE MEDICINE USES OLIVE SOUP AS A SORE-THROAT RECIPE – THE ONLY OCCURRENCE OF THE OLIVE IN CHINESE CUISINE.

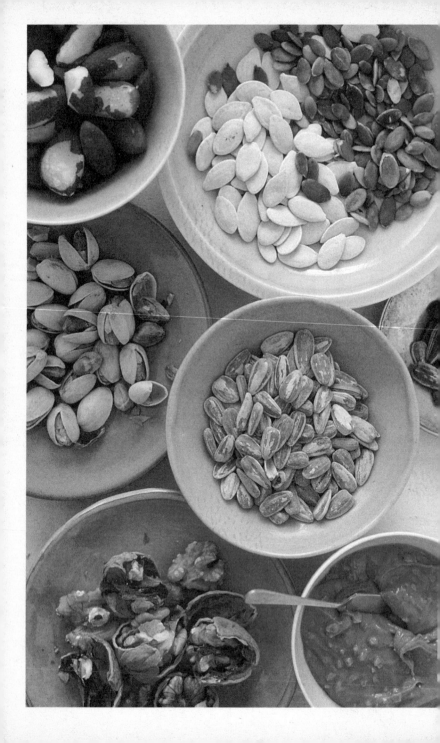

3. Nuts and Seeds

THESE MUFAS HAVE long been revered for their high levels of protein, fibre and antioxidants (not to mention those healthy fats!). Sprinkle on yogurt, cereal and salads; use as a topping for fish and chicken; or just snack on them by the handful.

HOW TO BUY AND USE: Nuts and seeds are sold in a variety of ways, including vacuum-sealed tins, glass jars, sealed bags and in bulk. They can be whole, sliced or chopped; raw or roasted; in or out of the shell. If purchasing in bulk, select a market that has a high turnover and uses covered bins so they'll be perfectly fresh. Unshelled nuts should be free from cracks or holes, feel somewhat heavy for their size and not rattle in the shell. Shelled nuts should be plump and look uniform in size and shape.

HOW TO STORE: Due to their high fat content, nuts and seeds tend to go rancid quickly once their shells are removed, especially if they're exposed to heat, light and humidity during storage, so buy them as fresh as possible. When kept in a cool, dry place in an airtight container, raw, unshelled nuts will keep from 6 months to a year, while shelled nuts will stay fresh for 3 to 4 months under the same conditions. Shelled nuts can be stored for 4 months in a refrigerator and 6 months in a freezer.

HISTORY

Nuts and seeds have a long, extensive history. Almonds were prized by Egypt's pharaohs. The use of flaxseed (linseed) goes as far back as the Stone Age and ancient Greece. Native Americans have been using sunflower seeds for more than 5,000 years and peanuts were a staple of the Aztec diet.

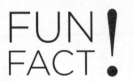

FUN FACT !

MACADAMIA NUTS PROVIDE MORE MUFA THAN ANY OTHER NUT OR SEED.

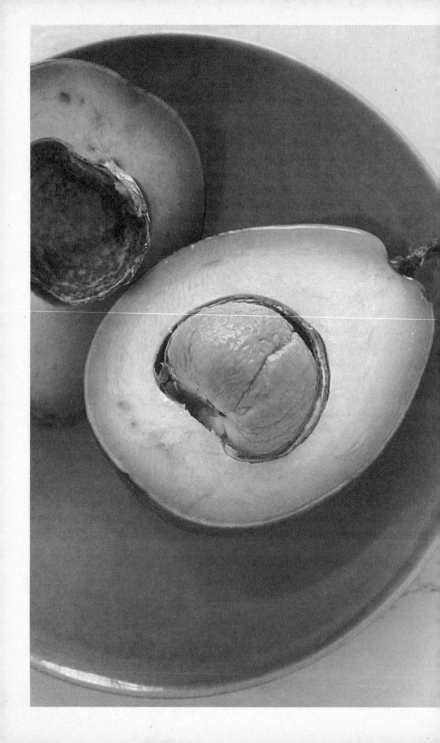

4. Avocados

ONCE A LUXURY FOOD reserved for royalty, super-creamy avocado is a feast of riches. Delicious mashed into a dip or sliced onto a salad, this MUFA is like butter, only better.

HOW TO BUY AND USE: When selecting any avocado, look for a fruit with slightly soft skin that yields slightly when you press it with your thumb. Avoid bruised, cracked or indented fruit. Those with teardrop-shaped necks have usually been tree ripened and will have a richer taste than rounded specimens. Once it's ripe, use a sharp knife to slice it lengthways, guiding the knife gently around the stone. Then twist the two halves against each other in opposite directions to separate. The stone will still be lodged in one half. Carefully nudge the knife into the stone and twist it out to discard. You can either gently peel away the skin or carefully score the avocado while still in the peel, cutting into long slices or chunks, and use a spoon to separate it from the skin.

HOW TO STORE: A whole, ripe avocado with the skin on will keep in the refrigerator for a day or two. A slightly unripe avocado can be ripened in just a day or two by storing it in a paper bag and keeping it on the kitchen counter. To prevent a leftover portion from browning, coat the exposed flesh with lemon juice, wrap tightly in clingfilm, and store in the refrigerator.

HISTORY

Avocados have been cultivated in South and Central America since 8000 BC. They were introduced to the United States in the early 20th century, when they were first planted in California and Florida.

FUN FACT!

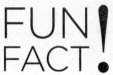

KNOBBLY HASS AVOCADOS HAVE A MUCH CREAMIER CONSISTENCY THAN THEIR SMOOTH FLORIDA COUNTERPARTS AND PROVIDE ALMOST TWICE THE MUFA PER SERVING.

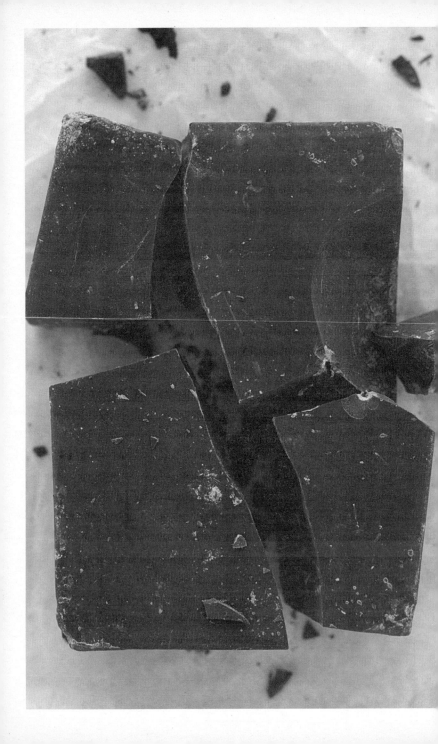

5. Dark Chocolate

OUR MOST BELOVED MUFA. The one that makes us swoon. The one that makes every meal or snack a little bit sweeter. And the one that makes everyone want to start the *Flat Belly Diet* – and never stop.

HOW TO BUY AND USE: Dark chocolate is low enough in sugar and high enough in monounsaturated fats to get the MUFA accolade in our book. Chocolate with a higher 'cacao', or cocoa content – the packet usually lists the percentage – is typically darker, less sweet and slightly more bitter, but in a good way. If you're used to milk chocolate, go dark gradually so you train your tastebuds to appreciate the stronger flavour of real, dark chocolate. You can buy chocolate in large chunks (popular with the baking set), as moulded bars or in chip form. I like chips because they're so easy to measure and use. (And when I want chocolate, I don't want to mess about with a knife and a grater!)

HOW TO STORE: Keep dark chocolate that's in its original sealed packet in a cool dry place (15.5–24°C/60–75°F). Once opened, chocolate should be transferred to an airtight container or bag and kept in the fridge (good) or freezer (best). During prolonged storage, chocolate will often 'bloom', or develop a white blush. It's perfectly safe to eat, though not very appetizing to look at. One solution: melt it – the bloom will disappear.

HISTORY

You're not the only one who loves chocolate. The ancient Mayans and Aztecs touted it as a food of the gods – and it's been a culinary mainstay ever since.

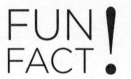

FUN FACT ! CHOCOLATE REALLY DOES MELT IN YOUR MOUTH BECAUSE ITS MELTING POINT IS SLIGHTLY BELOW HUMAN BODY TEMPERATURE.

READ A FLAT BELLY
SUCCESS
STORY

Kevin Martin

AGE: 50

POUNDS LOST:

13.5

IN 32 DAYS

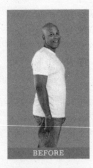
BEFORE

ALL-OVER INCHES LOST:

11.5

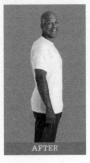
AFTER

IT'S NOT LIKE I DIDN'T CONTRIB-
UTE TO THIS BELLY,' LAMENTS
Kevin Martin. 'I'm a supervisor. So I ride
around all day in my van. You know
how that is. You spend your day eating
lots and lots of stuff that's not good for
you. I'd head out to work at 6 a.m., and
I'd stop on the way and get my coffee,
and I might get two doughnuts to go
with it. By nine, I'm getting a bacon,
egg and cheese sandwich and a Sunny
Delight. That's breakfast. By midday,
I'm eating pizza or a huge sandwich,
and that keeps me going until two,
when it's time for a couple of packets
of crisps and a drink. At four, I get
home and go straight for the biscuits in
the cupboard, and then it's dinnertime.'
After dinner, it's poker on the computer. The next day? 'Same thing all
over again.' After a long pause, he asks:
'Is it any wonder that spare tyre around
my waist was slowly inflating?

'I wanted to lose 12 to 15 pounds
and get rid of that spare tyre,' says the
50-year-old, adding that he's never
been on a diet before – not successfully,
anyway. He tried them several times
with his wife but never stayed on one
for more than a couple of days.

This time, he says, was different. 'I
guess the timing was just right with this
one. Summer was coming. And I
wanted to be able to take off my shirt

in public.' He also knew he needed something to get him off the computer – playing online poker had become his nightly activity – and into the gym. 'I belonged to a gym but never went. I was paying all that money for nothing. So because I was also on the [Flat Belly] exercise programme, I started going to the gym again.'

Kevin admits that the first 4 days – the Anti-Bloat Jumpstart – were a challenge for him. Going cold turkey from coffee was hard enough, he recollects. But giving up all the junk food? That was *really* hard for him. Still, he was committed. And he stuck to it. What kept him going was his athlete's sensibility. 'I wanted to finish it. Get to day 32. I knew I would, too. I used to be an athlete, and I played all kinds of sports. When you're an athlete, if you start something, you finish it.'

After the first full week, he was amazed at how great he was beginning to feel. He's happy he's doing something productive for himself *and* his body. Now when he gets home from work, instead of going for the biscuits and the computer, he heads for the gym or takes a ride on his bike – or sometimes both. He has the energy now, he says. 'I feel a lot better. I'm not tired ever – or hungry. My main objective was to be able to take my shirt off in public, and I'm there. Now that I've lost all this weight, I realize how terribly I had been treating my body. I won't be doing *that* again,' he says. 'Ever.'

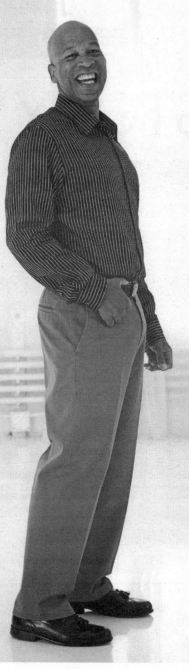

7

THE FOUR-WEEK PLAN:
QUICK-AND-EASY MEALS

UNLIKE MOST OTHER diets, the *Flat Belly Diet* doesn't require you to follow a day-by-day, meal-by-meal menu. Hooray! Instead, you will have a prescribed schedule of meals (four per day, including a Snack Pack) and a predetermined calorie count per meal and snack (roughly 400). Beyond that, we don't dictate what to eat when. Instead, we offer suggestions – and lots of them. *All of the meals are interchangeable*, so you can mix and match all you want. Our test panellists happily reported that this freedom of choice made it a breeze for them to follow the plan faithfully – even beyond the 4-week test period.

Remember, you will eat four 400-calorie meals each day: three meals plus one Snack Pack. Meals are categorized here as breakfast, lunch and dinner, but because every single one follows the *Flat Belly* '400 calories with a MUFA' rule, you can shuffle them however you like. If you want Pineapple-Ham Pizza for breakfast and Granola for dinner, go for it! There are 14 breakfasts and 28 lunches and dinners, so, if you like, you can go for maximum variety and have something different for every meal, every day, for 4 weeks. On the other hand, if you find one breakfast you love and want to make it part of your morning routine every day, that's fine, too. (Join the creature-of-habit club. I've eaten the same breakfast every day for 3 years!) For leisurely days when you have more time on your hands and feel like cooking, turn to Chapter 8, where you'll find more than 80 fabulous *Flat Belly Diet* recipes.

You may be tempted to create your own meals from the start, but we caution you against this, at least for the first 28 days. It's important for you to get into the rhythm of the *Flat Belly Diet* way of eating first. Once you are fully acquainted with the portion sizes, MUFA servings and basic composition of the meals, feel free to create your own meals as often as you like. However, customizing the meals to your taste is easy. The two questions below will clarify the most important points for you to keep in mind when altering the meals in this chapter.

The Food Questions

Can I swap around the ingredients in a meal?

Yes and no. You should not move items from one meal to another – that is, you can't delete your MUFA from breakfast and add it to lunch. But you *can* swap around foods within a meal, as long as:

■ they're within the same food group, such as tomatoes and red peppers or turkey and chicken; and

■ the food you added provides about the same number of calories as the food you took out. The calories for each ingredient appear in parentheses.

Do I have to buy the suggested brand?

Cynthia selected particular brands because of their taste, quality, availability and, most importantly, nutritional value. The nutritional quality of foods in certain categories varies widely, so she scoured the supermarket aisles, read countless labels and hand-picked the high-quality brands that met her tough nutritional standards. Including these foods guarantees steady weight loss because their precise calorie level per serving has been incorporated into the plan. So, yes, I encourage you to use these brands. However, if you can't or prefer not to, simply replace them with comparable foods with as close to the same calorie levels.

Flat Belly Breakfasts

Among our testers – and their families! – the Peachy Pecan Oatmeal on the next page was a huge hit. MUFAs are in **bold**, and ingredient calorie counts are in parentheses.

Apple–Almond Oatmeal: 1
packet Oats So Simple® original variety made up with 180ml (6 fl oz) semi-skimmed milk (180) mixed with 1 apple, sliced (80), and sprinkled with a pinch of mixed spice and 2tbsp chopped or flaked **almonds** (109)
▓ Total Calories = 370

Banana–Pecan Oatmeal:
1 packet Oats So Simple® original variety made with 180ml (6 fl oz) semi-skimmed milk (180) mixed with 1 large sliced banana (100) and sprinkled with cinnamon, nutmeg, and 2tbsp **pecans** (90)
▓ Total Calories = 370

Banana Split Oatmeal: 1 packet
Oats So Simple® original variety made up with 180ml (6 fl oz) semi-skimmed milk (180) mixed with 3tbsp fresh strawberries or 3tbsp microwaved frozen berries (50) and topped with ½ small sliced banana (35), 10g/½oz dark chocolate chips (50), and 2tbsp **peanuts** (110)
▓ Total Calories = 425

Blueberry–Nut Oatmeal:
1 packet Oats So Simple® apple and blueberry variety made up with 180ml (6 fl oz) semi-skimmed milk (215) mixed with

3tbsp fresh or frozen blueberries, warmed in microwave for 1 minute (50), and 2tbsp **cashews** (100)
▓ Total Calories = 365

Raisin Toast: 2 medium slices raisin
bread, toasted (200), spread with 30g/1oz low-fat soft cheese (50) and topped with 2tbsp **walnuts** (82); 1 medium apple (80)
▓ Total Calories = 412

Fruit & Nut Cereal: 1 serving (16g)
whole grain puffed wheat with 120ml (4fl oz) semi-skimmed milk (120), 2tbsp **almonds** (109), and 8 dried apricots (98)
▓ Total Calories = 327

Mediterranean BLT: 1 whole wheat
English muffin, toasted (130), spread with 2tbsp **black olive tapenade** (88) and 1 light Mini Babybel cheese (42); add 5 slices cucumber (5), 3 sun-dried tomatoes jarred in olive oil (30), 3 large lettuce leaves (3), and 2 small slices grilled lean back bacon (90)
▓ Total Calories = 388

Muesli & Yogurt: 4tbsp low-sugar
muesli (220) mixed with 1 fat-free/light vanilla yogurt with no artificial sweeteners

(200g/7oz) (100) and 1tbsp **almonds** (55);
20 seedless red grapes (60)
■ **Total Calories = 435**

PB&B: 1 whole wheat English muffin,
toasted (130), spread with 2tbsp natural
unsalted **peanut butter** (190) and topped
with 1 small sliced banana (70)
■ **Total Calories = 390**

Peachy Pecan Oatmeal: 1 packet
Oats So Simple® original variety made up
with 180ml (6 fl oz) semi-skimmed milk
(180) mixed with 1 fresh sliced peach (60)
or 6 slices tinned peaches in natural juice
drained (60) and sprinkled with nutmeg
and 2tbsp **pecans** (90)
■ **Total Calories = 330**

Peanut Butter Toast & Yogurt:
1 medium slice seeded bread, toasted (80),
spread with 2tbsp natural creamy **peanut
butter** (190); 1 fat-free/light vanilla yogurt

(200g/7oz) (100)
■ **Total Calories = 370**

Pecan Raisin Cereal: 1 serving
(16g) whole grain puffed wheat with 120ml
(4fl oz) semi-skimmed milk (120) sprinkled
with 2tbsp **pecans** (90) and 3tbsp raisins
(98)
■ **Total Calories = 308**

Vanilla Macadamia Parfait:
4tbsp low-sugar muesli (200) mixed with 1
fat-free/light vanilla yogurt with no
artificial sweeteners (200g/7oz) (100)
topped with 2tbsp **macadamia nuts** (120)
■ **Total Calories = 420**

Egg and Avocado Muffin:
1 whole wheat English muffin, toasted
(130), topped with 2 poached eggs (150)
and 1 sliced tomato (10) and 60g/2oz
sliced Hass **avocado** (96)
■ **Total Calories = 386**

SASS FROM SASS

'Why So Many Calorie Counts?'

The numbers in the parentheses correspond to the
calorie content of each ingredient. I provide them for a
few reasons: first, to help you become familiar with the
calorie levels of various ingredients – you may be sur-
prised to find out just how many or few calories there
are in certain foods. The second reason is to help you
customize the plan. If you dislike a certain ingredient,
don't have the same brand on hand, want to use up
something you already have or want to experiment
with a different way of preparing a meal, you can. Just
be sure the food you added provides about the same
number of calories as the one you took away. Use the
nutrition information on the label to check the calorie
content of packaged foods.   – *Cynthia*

Flat Belly Lunches

My favourite lunchbox standby: the Dijon Turkey Wrap on the next page. Yum! As with the breakfasts, MUFAs are in **bold**, and ingredient calorie counts are in parentheses.

Chicken Tacos: 1 large seeded tortilla wrap, warmed (180), filled evenly with 50g/1³/₄oz cooked cold chicken breast (60), and topped with small handful of fresh baby spinach leaves (3), ½ pot salsa (50) and 60g/2oz sliced Hass **avocado** (96)
▦ Total Calories = 389

California Chicken Burger:

1 grilled medium chicken breast (100g/3½oz), skinless (120) on 1 small seeded wholemeal bap (130), dressed with 1tbsp Dijon mustard (0), 3 large lettuce leaves (3), 30g/1oz roasted red peppers (jarred in water) (30), and 60g/2oz sliced Hass **avocado** (96)
▦ Total Calories = 379

Chicken Lettuce Wraps I:

100g/3½oz grilled chicken breast (120), glazed with 2tbsp (30g) reduced-fat mayonnaise (80) and wrapped in 4 large lettuce leaves (4); 3tbsp fresh mangetout (20) with 1tbsp reduced-fat hummus (60) sprinkled with 2tbsp **pine nuts** (113), for dipping
▦ Total Calories = 393

Chicken Lettuce Wraps II:

100g/3½oz grilled chicken breast (120), chilled, topped with 1tbsp **pesto sauce** (80), 30g/1oz roasted red peppers (jarred) (30) and 60g/2oz fresh mozzarella (160) wrapped

in 4 large romaine lettuce leaves (4)
▦ Total Calories = 394

Cheesy Spinach Pasta:

130g/4½oz cooked weight whole wheat penne pasta (140) tossed with 1tbsp **olive oil** (119), 2tbsp fresh grated Parmesan cheese (40), small handful of fresh baby spinach leaves (3), 2tbsp sliced spring onions (6), and 150g/5½oz of tomato pasta sauce (60)
▦ Total Calories = 368

Chilled Chicken Pasta:

130g/4½oz cooked weight whole wheat penne pasta (140) tossed with 1tbsp **pesto sauce** (80), 90g/3oz pre-cooked chicken breast, diced (90), 12 cherry tomatoes, halved (30), 2tbsp grated carrots (15), and 1tbsp fresh grated Parmesan cheese (20)
▦ Total Calories = 375

Chilled Spicy Sausage Pasta:

50g/1³/₄oz cooked extra-lean/low-fat pork sausages, chopped (150), tossed with 130g/4½oz cooked weight whole wheat penne pasta (140), 12 cherry tomatoes, halved (30), 2tbsp grated carrot (15), 2 sticks chopped celery (5) with 1tbsp **pesto sauce** (80)
▦ Total Calories = 420

Crunchy Tuna Melt: 1 medium slice seeded bread (80) topped with 100g/3½oz

SASS FROM SASS

What about alcohol?

Whether or not you drink on the *Flat Belly Diet* is up to you. As a health care professional, my goal has always been to help people make informed decisions that work best for their own lives. So here's the information I always give regarding alcohol: current dietary guidelines recommend that if you don't drink, you should not start. In moderation, alcohol has been shown to lower the risk of heart disease, but it also carries risks. Just one drink a day is linked to an increased risk of breast cancer, and more-than-moderate drinking is tied to cirrhosis of the liver, high blood pressure, cancers of the upper gastro-intestinal tract, stroke, injuries and violence.

Some people are advised not to consume alcoholic beverages at all, including pregnant and breastfeeding women and individuals taking medications that can interact with alcohol.

That said, most adults do consume alcohol, so if you do already drink, practise moderation, meaning no more than 2 to 3 units of alcohol per day for women, and 3 to 4 for men. (One unit is equal to a pub measure of spirits, ½ pint of beer and there are 2.3 units in a 175-ml glass of white or red wine.) Each unit contains around 100 calories, so to stay on track with the *Flat Belly Diet,* you'll need to balance out those calories somehow. You can either burn 100 extra calories by exercising or shave 25 calories from each of your four meals – or 50 each from two. Taking 100 calories out of a single 400-calorie meal can leave you feeling too hungry, and since alcohol is an appetite stimulant, that could be a recipe for overeating.   – *Cynthia*

water-packed tuna (100), 2tbsp **sunflower seeds** (90), and 1 slice half-fat Cheddar cheese (80), then placed under grill or in toaster oven to melt
■ Total Calories = 350

Dijon Turkey Wrap: 1 large seeded tortilla wrap, warmed (180) spread with 1tbsp Dijon mustard (0), sprinkled

with 2tbsp **pumpkin seeds** (148), and filled with 50g/1¾oz cooked wafer-thin turkey breast (50), ¼ of a sliced red onion (15), ½ fresh plum tomato, sliced (6), and 3 large lettuce leaves (3)
■ Total Calories = 402

Dipping Trio: 2tbsp frozen thawed or fresh edamame beans (120), dressed with fat-free French dressing; 3 Ryvita® dark rye crispbread crackers (60); 5 baby carrots (25) with 2tbsp tahini for dipping (178)

■ **Total Calories = 383**

Turkey and Avocado Roll-Ups:
100g/3¹/₂oz smoked turkey slices (100) wrapped around 1 pot (113g) reduced-fat guacamole (140), 50g/1³/₄oz sliced roasted red peppers (jarred in water) (50), and 2tbsp **pine nuts** (113)

■ **Total Calories = 403**

Ham & Blue Cheese Salad:
4 small handfuls of baby leaf spinach (12) tossed with 2tbsp fat-free French dressing (0) and topped with ¹/₂ fresh plum tomato, sliced (6), 100g/3¹/₂oz wafer-thin ham, chopped (100), 30g/1oz crumbled Gorgonzola (100), and 2tbsp **pumpkin seeds** (148)

■ **Total Calories = 366**

Spicy Sausage Wraps:
Sauté in 1tbsp **rapeseed (canola) oil** (124): 50g/1³/₄oz cooked extra-lean/low-fat pork sausages, chopped (150), ¹/₂ a fresh chopped red pepper (25) and ¹/₂ a sliced red onion (30); spread evenly onto 4 large lettuce leaves (4), sprinkle with 30g/1oz crumbled Gorgonzola (100), and roll up

■ **Total Calories = 433**

SASS FROM SASS

'Take a Lunch Break!'

A recent survey found that a whopping 74 per cent of American office workers eat lunch at their desks. Eating while working can cause you to eat too fast, lose track of how much you've eaten and distract you from the taste and enjoyment of your meal. Follow these lunchtime rules to help make your midday meal a priority.

■ Set your mobile phone or computer alarm to remind you to stop and eat. When it goes off, don't hit the snooze or dismiss it. You can pick up where you left off after your meal, feeling re-energized.

■ Commit to eating lunch with a colleague. When you know a friend is waiting for you, you won't talk yourself into staying at your desk.

■ Use real plates and cutlery. People in France, Greece, Italy, Portugal, Spain and other countries in Europe (where the average lunchtime is 50 per cent longer but waistlines are smaller) rely on this tradition to make each meal feel special. Keep a set in your office kitchen – washing them up will add just a few seconds onto your meal.

■ If you really have to eat at your desk, try not to work while you eat. Take a few deep breaths, and savour every bite – even if it's only for 10 minutes.   – *Cynthia*

Falafel Pitta Pocket: 1 wholemeal pitta toasted (160) filled with 2 mini falafel (100) and drizzled with 1tbsp **olive oil** (119); 50g/1³/₄oz tzatziki for dipping (70)
▤ **Total Calories = 449**

Mediterranean Wrap: 1 large seeded tortilla wrap warmed (180) spread with 2tbsp **black olive tapenade** (88) and filled with 50g/1³/₄oz turkey ham (50), ½ a sliced red onion (30); ½ fresh plum tomato, sliced (6), and 3 large lettuce leaves (3)
▤ **Total Calories = 357**

Cheese and Turkey Wrap:
1 large seeded tortilla wrap warmed (180) spread with 2tbsp **black olive tapenade** (88) and filled with 50g/1³/₄oz cooked turkey breast (50), 1 slice half-fat Cheddar (30g/1oz) (80), 2 sticks chopped celery (5), and 3 large lettuce leaves (3)
▤ **Total Calories = 406**

Niçoise Salad: 130g/4½oz mixed baby salad leaves (15) tossed with Dijon mustard to coat (0) and topped with 100g/3½oz new potatoes, cubed, boiled and chilled (75), 10 sliced large **black olives** (50), 2tbsp cooked gréen beans (25), 2 sticks chopped celery (5), 6 cherry tomato halves (15) and 100g/3½oz water-packed tuna (100) and 1 hard-boiled egg sliced (75)
▤ **Total Calories = 360**

Pesto, Ham & Cheese Sandwich: 1 whole wheat English muffin (130) spread with 1tbsp **pesto sauce** (80) and filled with 50g/1³/₄oz cooked ham (50), ½ fresh plum tomato, sliced (6), 3 large lettuce leaves (3), and 1 slice half-fat Cheddar cheese (80); 6 cherry tomato halves (15)
▤ **Total Calories = 364**

Picnic Lunch: 4 Ryvita® dark rye crispbread crackers (120) spread with Dijon mustard (0), 5 turkey slices (75g/2½oz) (70), 10 large **green olives** (50), and 5 baby carrots (25) with ¼ pot reduced-fat hummus (120) for dipping
▤ **Total Calories = 385**

Prawn Lettuce Wraps: 4 large lettuce leaves (4) filled evenly with 100g/3½oz cooked prawns (100), mixed with 2tbsp (30g) reduced-fat mayonnaise (80) and tossed with 2 sticks chopped celery (5), ¼ minced red onion (15), a fresh chopped red pepper (25), and 2tbsp **cashews** (100); 1 orange (62)
▤ **Total Calories = 391**

Chicken Pitta Melt: ½ large wholemeal pitta (80) toasted and filled with 1 slice half-fat Cheddar cheese (80) and 1 medium (100g/3½oz) chicken breast without skin, grilled and sliced (120) and dressed with 3 large lettuce leaves (3), ½ fresh plum tomato, sliced (6), 60g/2oz sliced Hass **avocado** (96) and 2tbsp sliced onions (6)
▤ **Total Calories = 391**

Spicy Chicken Burger:
1 small seeded wholemeal bap (130), filled with 1 grilled medium (100g/3½oz) chicken breast, sliced, without skin (120), topped with 60g/2oz sliced Hass **avocado** (96), 2tbsp sliced onions (6), 1 sliced chilli pepper (4) and 1tbsp salsa (25)
▤ **Total Calories = 381**

Spaghetti & Tomato Sauce:

130g/4½oz cooked weight whole wheat spaghetti (140) tossed with 1tbsp **olive oil** (119) and topped with 2tbsp tomato pasta sauce (60) and 2tbsp fresh grated Parmesan cheese (80)

▨ **Total Calories = 399**

Spinach Chicken Wrap:

1 large seeded tortilla wrap warmed (180) filled with 1 grilled medium (100g/3½oz) chicken breast without skin, sliced (120), and topped with 1 small handful fresh baby spinach leaves (3), 2tbsp chopped spring onions (4) and 60g/2oz sliced Hass **avocado** (96)

▨ **Total Calories = 403**

Tuna Pitta: ½ a wholemeal pitta (80)

filled with 100g/3½oz water-packed tuna (100), 2 diced sun-dried tomatoes jarred in extra virgin olive oil (20), 2tbsp chopped **walnuts** (82), and 30g/1oz crumbled feta cheese (80)

▨ **Total Calories = 362**

Tuna Salad: 130g/4½oz mixed baby

salad leaves (15) tossed with 2tbsp low-fat vinaigrette (45) and topped with 100g/3½oz water-packed tuna (100), 2tbsp **walnuts** (82), and 30g/1oz crumbled feta cheese (80); 1 plum (25)

▨ **Total Calories = 347**

Turkey Cranberry Muffin:

1 whole wheat English muffin (130) spread with 1 wedge of Laughing Cow® Light reduced-fat cheese spread (25) and filled with 75g/2½oz cold cooked turkey breast (75), 1tbsp dried cranberries (45), and 2tbsp **walnuts** (82)

▨ **Total Calories = 357**

Waldorf Pitta: 1 wholemeal pitta

(160) spread with 2 wedges Laughing Cow® Light reduced-fat cheese spread (50) and filled with 2 sticks chopped celery (5), 1 medium apple, sliced (80), 2tbsp **walnuts** (82), and 3 large lettuce leaves (3)

▨ **Total Calories = 380**

SASS FROM SASS

'The Cure for After-Work Munchies'

Many of the women I've advised who work away from home eat lunch between noon and 1 p.m. but don't even start making dinner until well after 6 p.m. That means their hunger signals are in high gear before they even set foot in the kitchen – a perfect recipe for munching on pre-dinner snacks like crackers, crisps or cheese or nibbling on meal ingredients while cooking. The best fix is to plan your Snack Pack in between lunch and dinner, around 3 or 4 p.m. The MUFA from your Snack Pack will help you stay full and satisfied, so you'll still feel energized (and even-tempered) when you start cooking. And because you won't be so ravenous, you won't rush through your meal preparation. – *Cynthia*

Flat Belly Dinners

Don't hesitate to make additional portions of these dinners for your family. Our testers raved and were so thankful that these options pleased husbands, kids and teenagers alike! As with breakfasts and lunches, MUFAs are in **bold**, and ingredient calorie counts are in parentheses.

California Turkey Salad:

130g/4½oz mixed baby salad leaves (15) tossed with 2tbsp light balsamic vinaigrette (45) and topped with 30g/1oz crumbled Gorgonzola (100), and 2tbsp **walnuts** (82); 1 small pear (50)

▓ **Total Calories = 367**

Cheesy Veggie Pasta: 3 rings red

pepper chopped (10), 2 broccoli florets (20), and 2tbsp sliced onions (6) sautéed in 1tbsp **olive oil** (119) and tossed with 50g/1¾oz ricotta cheese (70), 1tbsp fresh grated Parmesan cheese (40) and 130g/4½oz cooked weight whole wheat penne pasta (140)

▓ **Total Calories = 405**

Chicago-style Hot Dog: 1 small

50g/2oz hot dog sausage (80), browned in frying pan in 1tbsp **peanut (groundnut) oil** (119), on 1 hot dog roll (140) dressed with 1tbsp mustard (0), 2tbsp diced onions (6), 2tbsp sweet hot dog relish (30), ½ fresh tomato, diced (6), and a dash of celery seed

▓ **Total Calories = 381**

Chicken Caesar: 130g/4½oz mixed

baby salad leaves (15) tossed with 1tbsp **olive oil** (119) and 1tbsp low-fat Caesar dressing (30) and topped with 100g/3½oz pre-cooked chicken breast (120), chilled (optional: sear on grill); 25g/1oz sliced Parmesan cheese (104); and 1 Ryvita® dark rye crispbread cracker (30)

▓ **Total Calories = 418**

Chicken Caprese: 50g/1¾oz

organic grilled chicken breast (60) served with 3tbsp cooked wild rice (150) and tomato mozzarella salad made with 1 plum tomato, sliced (12), 1oz sliced reduced-fat mozzarella (50), and 2 fresh basil leaves (0) drizzled with 1tbsp **olive oil** (119) and 1tbsp balsamic vinegar (5), and dusted with cracked black pepper

▓ **Total Calories = 406**

Edamame Bean Salad: 130g/4½oz

mixed baby salad leaves (15) tossed with 2tbsp low-fat salad dressing (30) and topped with 3tbsp edamame, fresh or frozen and thawed (180), 130g/4½oz canned mandarin oranges, drained (50), and 2tbsp **almonds** (109)

▓ **Total Calories = 384**

Edamame Bean and Rice Salad:
2tbsp cooked rice (100), chilled, tossed with 2tbsp edamame, fresh or frozen and thawed (120), 3tbsp mixed stir-fry vegetables (25), 2tbsp low-fat salad dressing (30) and 2tbsp **cashews** (100)
▧ Total Calories = 355

Grilled Chicken Salad:
130g/4¹/₂oz mixed baby salad leaves (15) tossed with 2tbsp balsamic vinegar (10) and 1tbsp **olive oil** (119) and topped with 100g/3¹/₂oz grilled chicken breast (120), 2 broccoli florets (20), 2tbsp grated carrots (15), ¹/₄ sliced red onion (15), 3tbsp sweet corn, frozen or tinned (100), and freshly ground black pepper
▧ Total Calories = 414

Grilled Pork Salad:
100g/3¹/₂oz pork tenderloin, grilled (120), served on a bed of 130g/4¹/₂oz mixed baby salad leaves (15) tossed with 130g/4¹/₂oz drained pineapple pieces (60), 2 rings chopped red pepper (10), 30g/1oz crumbled feta (80), 2tbsp balsamic vinegar (10), and 1tbsp **olive oil** (119)
▧ Total Calories = 414

Mexican Salad:
130g/4¹/₂oz mixed baby salad leaves (15) topped with 100g/3¹/₂oz refried beans (90), 3tbsp sweet corn, frozen thawed or tinned (100), ¹/₄ sliced red onion (15), 1tbsp salsa (50), and 60g/2oz sliced Hass **avocado** (96)
▧ Total Calories = 366

Pepperoni Pizza:
1 flat wholemeal pitta (160) brushed on one side with 1tbsp **olive oil** (119) and topped with 1tbsp tomato pasta sauce (30), 2 lunch box mini reduced-fat Peperami sausages sliced (76), and 15g/¹/₂oz half-fat grated cheese (35); warm under grill to heat through
▧ Total Calories = 420

Pineapple-Ham Pizza:
1 flat wholemeal pitta (160) brushed on one side with 1tbsp **olive oil** (119) and topped with 1tbsp tomato pasta sauce (30), 60g/2oz drained pineapple pieces (30), 2 rings fresh chopped red pepper (10), 50g/1³/₄oz cooked cold sliced ham, chopped (50), and 15g/¹/₂oz crumbled Gorgonzola (50); warm under grill to heat through
▧ Total Calories = 449

Pork with Stir-Fry Vegetables:
6tbsp mixed stir-fry vegetables (50), sautéed in 1tbsp **rapeseed (canola) oil** (124) flavoured with ground peppercorns and served with 100g/3¹/₂oz pork tenderloin, sliced (120), and 60g/2oz cooked brown rice (110)
▧ Total Calories = 404

Ricotta Calzone:
50g/1³/₄oz ricotta cheese (70), mixed with 2 sun-dried tomatoes jarred in olive oil, diced (20), 1tbsp **olive oil** (119), 1tsp minced garlic (10), and 4 fresh basil leaves, sliced (0), and stuffed into 1 wholemeal pitta (160); warm under grill until pitta is golden and cheese is bubbly; serve with 1tbsp fresh tomato pasta sauce (30) for dipping
▧ Total Calories = 409

Salmon Pistachio Lettuce Wraps:
4 large lettuce leaves (4) filled evenly with 1tbsp reduced-fat hummus (120), 100g/3½oz tinned salmon (150), ½ fresh plum tomato, diced (6), 2tbsp diced cucumber (5), and 2tbsp **pistachios** (88)
▓ Total Calories = 367

Salmon Sandwich:
2 slices seeded whole grain bread (160) spread with 2tbsp **black olive tapenade** (88), 100g/3½oz tinned salmon (150), ½ fresh plum tomato, diced (6), and 2 large lettuce leaves (2)
▓ Total Calories = 406

Salmon Steak Almondine:
130g/4½oz grilled salmon steak (215) served with 4tbsp cooked green beans steamed or microwaved (50), and dressed with freshly ground white pepper and 2tbsp sliced **almonds** (109)
▓ Total Calories = 374

Savoury Turkey Pasta:
2 broccoli florets (20) and 12 mini plum tomatoes, sliced (30), sautéed in 1tbsp **olive oil** (119) and tossed with 4 fresh basil leaves, sliced (0), 100g/3½oz dry-fried turkey mince (100), and 130g/4½oz cooked weight whole wheat penne pasta (140)
▓ Total Calories = 429

Sesame–Ginger Prawn Wrap:
1 large seeded tortilla wrap (180) filled with 100g/3½oz cooked prawns (100), 3tbsp mangetout (10), 2 sticks chopped celery (5), and 2tbsp **cashews** (100) and drizzled with 1tbsp fat-free sesame and ginger dressing (0)
▓ Total Calories = 395

Prawn and Mangetout Sesame Pasta:
50g/1¾oz cooked prawns (50), chilled, and 115g/4oz cooked weight whole wheat pasta spirals (140) tossed with 1tbsp **sesame oil** (120), 3tbsp mangetout (10), 2tbsp chopped spring onions (4), and 2 sticks chopped celery (5) and sprinkled with 1tbsp whole black sesame seeds (50)
▓ Total Calories = 379

Slaw Dog:
1 small 50g/1¾oz hot dog sausage (80) browned in frying pan in 1tbsp **peanut (groundnut) oil** (119), on 1 hot dog bun (140) dressed with 1tbsp mustard (0) and 1 heaped tbsp reduced-calorie coleslaw (50)
▓ Total Calories = 389

Spicy Prawns:
100g/3½oz cooked prawns (100), and 145g/5oz fresh asparagus spears (30) sautéed in 1tbsp **rapeseed (canola) oil** (124), 1tsp minced garlic jarred in water (10), 1tbsp fresh chopped parsley (0), and freshly ground black pepper served on 3tbsp cooked wild rice
▓ Total Calories = 404

Spinach Burrito:
1 large seeded tortilla wrap (180) filled with 1 small handful fresh spinach (3), 1tsp minced garlic (10), and ¼ of sliced red onion (15) sautéed in 1tbsp **olive oil** (119) and topped with 30g/1oz crumbled feta cheese (80)
▓ Total Calories = 407

Stir-Fried Chicken:
6tbsp mixed stir-fry vegetables (50), sautéed in 1tbsp **rapeseed (canola) oil** (124) flavoured with

ground peppercorns, served with 100g/3¹/₂oz organic grilled chicken breast (120) and 60g/2oz cooked brown rice (110)

▨ **Total Calories = 404**

Turkey Quesadilla: Spread 1 wedge Laughing Cow® Light reduced-fat cheese spread (25) on 1 large seeded tortilla wrap (18). On half of wrap, place 50g/1³/₄oz cooked turkey breast slices (50), 1 small handful baby spinach leaves (1), 30g/1oz crumbled feta (80), and 10 sliced large **black olives** (50). Fold over and heat in toaster oven or a non-stick pan over medium heat

▨ **Total Calories = 380**

Turkey Sauté: 5 rings fresh chopped red pepper (20) and ¹/₄ sliced red onion (15) sautéed in 1tbsp **olive oil** (119), tossed with 2 chopped spring onions (4), 4 fresh basil leaves, sliced (0), and 100g/3¹/₂oz

dry-fried turkey mince (100), served with 90g/3oz spicy potato wedges (180) cooked under grill or in oven

▨ **Total Calories = 438**

Turkey Tacos: Sauté 2 rings chopped red pepper (10) and 2tbsp sliced red onion (12) in 1tbsp **olive oil** (119). Brown 100g/3¹/₂oz dry-fried turkey mince (100). Fill 3 taco shells (150) evenly with turkey, then add pepper mixture and sprinkle with 2 chopped spring onions (4) and 2tbsp grated carrots (15)

▨ **Total Calories = 410**

Salmon Cashew Salad:
130g/4¹/₂oz mixed baby salad leaves (15) tossed with 2tbsp low-fat salad dressing (40) and topped with 130g/4¹/₂oz grilled salmon steak (215) and 2tbsp **cashews** (100)

▨ **Total Calories = 370**

SASS FROM SASS

'You Are Better Off with Breakfast!'

When I was a dietitian in private practice, at least once a week someone would tell me that they 'do better' when they skip breakfast. Unfortunately, this isn't true for anybody, and research proves it. In fact, a whopping 78 per cent of successful dieters registered with the US National Weight Control Registry, a database of individuals who've lost 30 pounds or more and have kept it off for at least a year, eat breakfast. What about the theory that skipping this meal is a natural way to eliminate calories? Studies show that those who skip breakfast make up for those calories by unknowingly eating more later in the day. Some of my clients swore that eating breakfast made them hungrier. Well, in fact, eating breakfast does stimulate your appetite because it kicks your metabolism into high gear. A faster metabolism means a flatter belly and more calories burned all day long, so overall, you are better off with breakfast.   – *Cynthia*

Snack Pack Options

There are 28 Snack Pack choices to select from. You will see 10 sweet options, 10 savoury, 4 grab-and-go choices and 4 smoothies. MUFAs are in **bold**.

YOU CAN HAVE ONE SNACK PACK to 'spend' per day.

PLAN YOUR SNACK PACK IN ADVANCE. I recommend carving out about 10 minutes each night to think through your schedule for the following day. You should decide where in the day you'll 'place' your Snack Pack based on what you have planned. You may need to pack it the night before and bring it with you so you'll have it ready when you need it.

YOU CAN EAT THE SNACK PACK either between breakfast and lunch, between lunch and dinner, or between dinner and bedtime – whichever is best for your schedule. I just ask that you use it to ensure that you do not go more than 4 hours without eating. The goal is to use the Snack Pack to keep your energy and blood sugar steady, keep your metabolism revved up, and prevent your hunger from getting out of control (which often results in rebound overeating).

Sweet Blueberry–Almond Oatmeal:

1 packet original Oats So Simple®, cooked with 180ml (6fl oz) semi-skimmed milk, topped with 3tbsp blueberries and 2tbsp **almonds**
▨ **Total Calories = 350**

Chocolate–Raspberry Oatmeal:

1 packet original Oats So Simple®, cooked, with 180ml (6fl oz) semi-skimmed milk topped with 3tbsp raspberries and 45g/1½oz **dark chocolate chips**
▨ **Total Calories = 440**

Tropical–Nut Oatmeal: 1 packet

original Oats So Simple®, cooked with 180ml (6fl oz) semi-skimmed milk topped with 130g/4½oz approx 3 rings tinned pineapple and 2tbsp **macadamia nuts**
▨ **Total Calories = 363**

PB&A Oatmeal: 2tbsp **peanut**

butter swirled into 1 packet original Oats So Simple®, cooked with 180ml (6fl oz) semi-skimmed milk, and topped with ½ medium sliced apple
▨ **Total Calories = 418**

Apple Snack: 1 medium apple cut

into wedges with 2tbsp **peanut butter** as a dip, and 30g/1oz plain popcorn
▨ **Total Calories = 370**

Pineapple 'Sundae': 130g/4½oz

(approx 3 rings) pineapple, tinned in pineapple juice, mixed into cottage cheese, low-fat 200g/7oz sprinkled with 2tbsp (6 halves) chopped **walnuts**
▨ **Total Calories = 350**

Strawberry–Chocolate 'Sundae': 3tbsp sliced strawberries and 45g/1½oz **dark chocolate chips** mixed into cottage cheese, low-fat 200g/7oz
■ **Total Calories = 420**

PB&A Muffin: 1 whole wheat English muffin spread with 2tbsp **peanut butter**, topped with 1 medium sliced apple
■ **Total Calories = 400**

Apples & Crackers: 3 Ryvita® crispbreads spread with 2tbsp **peanut butter**, topped or eaten with 1 medium sliced apple
■ **Total Calories = 360**

Berry–Nut Whip: 6tbsp sliced strawberries and 2tbsp **peanuts** mixed into 200g/7oz light vanilla yogurt
■ **Total Calories = 363**

Savoury

Hummus Dip: Reduced-fat hummus 100g/3½oz – sprinkled with 2tbsp **pine nuts** served with red pepper, sliced – 10 rings
■ **Total Calories = 393**

Deli Snack: 3 Ryvita® crispbread spread with 2tbsp **black olive tapenade**, cherry tomatoes (12) and cooked turkey breast slices – 100g/3½oz
■ **Total Calories = 320**

Cheesy Black Bean Dip:
Butter beans tinned, drained – 100g/3tbsp rinsed and mashed, topped with 60g/2oz chopped Hass **avocado**, and sprinkled with 2 chopped light cheese strings. Serve with 10 baby carrots
■ **Total Calories = 336**

Butter Bean Dip 'n' Tomatoes: tinned butter beans – 100g/3tbsp – rinsed, drained, mashed and mixed with cherry tomatoes (12) topped with 60g/2oz chopped Hass **avocado**, and sprinkled with 1 chopped string cheese and served with 3 Ryvita® crispbreads
■ **Total Calories = 356**

Open Turkey Sandwich: 1 whole wheat English muffin spread with 2tbsp **green olive tapenade**, topped with 100g/3½oz cooked cold turkey breast slices and artichoke hearts, tinned in water – 4 hearts, drained
■ **Total Calories = 380**

Open Tomato Sandwich:
1 whole wheat English muffin spread with cottage cheese, low-fat (200g/7oz) and cherry tomatoes (12) and sprinkled with 2tbsp **pine nuts**
■ **Total Calories = 433**

Cheese & Crispbreads: 100g/3½oz cottage cheese, low-fat, mixed with 10 rings chopped red pepper, pinch of Italian mixed herbs, and 10 sliced **black olives** served with 6 Ryvita® crispbreads
■ **Total Calories = 350**

Deli Wrap: 100g/3½oz cooked turkey breast slices filled with 1tbsp reduced-fat hummus, sprinkled with 2tbsp **pine nuts**, and rolled up
■ **Total Calories = 333**

Turkey Roll: 100g/3¹/₂oz cooked turkey breast slices filled with 60g/2oz chopped Hass **avocado**, 2 low-fat cheese strings chopped and red pepper, sliced – 10 rings and rolled up
▓ Total Calories = 336

Pesto Chicken Wrap: 100g/3¹/₂oz cooked chicken breast slices filled with mixture of cottage cheese, low-fat 100g/3¹/₂oz and 1tbsp **pesto**, topped with cherry tomatoes and artichoke hearts, tinned in water – 4 hearts, drained and rolled up
▓ Total Calories = 390

Grab & Go

Option 1: 2 low-fat cheese strings with pineapple, tinned in pineapple juice – 130g/4¹/₂oz (approx 3 rings) – baby carrots (10 carrots), and 2tbsp **peanuts**
▓ Total Calories = 320

Option 2: 2 low-fat cheese strings, popcorn – 30g/1oz plain or salt popped, 4tsp grated Parmesan, and 2tbsp **sunflower seeds**
▓ Total Calories = 370

Option 3: Fat-free/light fruit yogurt (200g/7oz), 1 medium apple, 2tbsp **Brazil nuts**, and 150 ml (5fl oz) semi-skimmed milk
▓ Total Calories = 360

Option 4: Fat-free/light fruit yogurt (200g/7oz), 1 medium orange, and 2tbsp **almonds**
▓ Total Calories = 279

Smoothies

Blueberry: Blend 150ml (5fl oz)semi-skimmed or half-fat soy milk, 1 fat-free/light vanilla yogurt (200g/7oz), and 3tbsp fresh blueberries plus a handful of ice OR 3tbsp frozen blueberries for 1 minute. Transfer to a glass, and stir in 1tbsp cold-pressed **flaxseed (linseed) oil**
▓ Total Calories = 360

Chocolate–Raspberry: Blend 150ml (5fl oz) semi-skimmed or half-fat soy milk, 1 fat-free/light vanilla yogurt (200g/7oz), 45g/1¹/₂oz dark **chocolate** chips and 3tbsp fresh raspberries plus a handful of ice OR 3tbsp frozen raspberries for 1 minute. Transfer to a glass, and eat with a spoon
▓ Total Calories = 440

Lemon: Blend 150ml (5fl oz) semi-skimmed or half-fat soy milk, 1 fat-free/light lemon yogurt (200g/7oz), 1 medium orange, sliced into sections, and a handful of ice for 1 minute. Transfer to a glass, and stir in 1tbsp cold-pressed **flaxseed (linseed) oil**
▓ Total Calories = 370

Apple Pie: Blend 150ml (5fl oz) semi-skimmed or half-fat soy milk, 1 fat-free/light vanilla yogurt (200g/7oz) , pinch of mixed spice, 1 medium apple, peeled, cored and chopped, 2tbsp smooth **peanut butter**, and a handful of ice for 1 minute. Transfer to a glass, and eat with a spoon
▓ Total Calories = 438

Create Your Own Snack Pack

KEEP THE TOTAL CALORIE COUNT UNDER 400, INCLUDE A SELECTION FROM THE MUFA LIST ON PAGE 101, AND PAIR WITH THE FOLLOWING FOODS.

SOME MUFA CHOICES:

- 10 olives (50)
- 190g/6½oz fresh or frozen soya (edamame) beans (244)
- 60g/2oz Hass avocado (96)
- 45g/1½oz dark chocolate chips (210)
- 2tbsp nuts or seeds (82-148)
- 2tbsp olive tapenade (88)
- 1tbsp rapeseed (canola) oil (124)

Please consult the full chart on page 101

GRAINS

½ large whole wheat tortilla wrap – 90 calories

Scotch pancakes – 1 – 65 calories

Raisin bread – 1 medium slice – 100 calories

Whole grain seeded bread – 1 medium slice – 80 calories

Puffed wheat cereal – 6tbsp – 80 calories

Frozen waffle – 1 – 100 calories

Oats So Simple® – 1 (27g/1oz) packet instant plain – 100 calories

Popcorn – 30g/1oz plain or salt – 100 calories

Ryvita® dark rye crisp-breads – 3 – 90 calories

Wholemeal pitta – ½ large – 80 calories

Whole wheat English muffin – 1 whole (75g/2½oz) – 130 calories

Microwaveable brown rice – ¼ pack – 100 calories

DAIRY

Half-fat Cheddar cheese slices – 1 slice (30g/1oz) – 80 calories

Reduced-fat Emmenthal cheese slices – 2 small slices (30g/1oz) – 70 calories

Cottage cheese, low-fat 200g/7oz – 160 calories

Feta cheese – 30g/1oz – 80 calories

Milk, semi-skimmed – 150ml – 70 calories

Cheese string, low-fat/light – 2 strings – 100 calories

Natural yogurt, low-fat (150g/5½oz) – 80 calories

Fat-free/light fruit yogurt (no artificial sweeten-ers), 200g/7oz – 100 calories

FRUITS

Apple, any variety, medium (size of a tennis ball) – 80 calories

Berries (blueberries, raspberries, or strawberries) – 3tbsp – 50 calories

Fresh cherries – 25 – 80 calories

Kiwi – 2 fruits – 100 calories

Mango – 150g/5½oz – 100 calories

Orange, medium – 70 calories

Papaya – ½ medium sized – 60 calories

Peach – 1 medium – 50 calories

Pear – 1 medium – 50 calories

Pineapple, canned in pineapple juice – 130g/4½ oz/approx 3 rings – 60 calories

Plums – 2 medium – 50 calories

Red or green grapes – 100g/3½oz/approx 20 grapes – 60 calories

Banana – 1 small – 70 calories

Unsweetened raisins – 2 small handfuls – 100 calories

Watermelon – 2 large slices – 70 calories

VEGETABLES

Artichoke hearts, tinned in water – 4 hearts – 50 calories

Baby carrots – 10 carrots – 50 calories

Broccoli florets, raw – 5 florets – 40 calories

Cauliflower florets, raw – 10 florets – 40 calories

Cherry tomatoes – 12 – 30 calories

Reduced-calorie coleslaw – 1 heaped tbsp – 50 calories

Tomato pasta sauce – 150g/5½oz – 70 calories

Mixed baby salad leaves – 130g/4½oz – 15 calories

Radishes – 20 large – 20 calories

Red pepper, sliced – 10 rings – 40 calories

Salsa – 100g/3½oz – 50 calories

PROTEINS

Lean wafer-thin ham – 100g/3½oz – 100 calories

Butter beans, tinned, drained – 100g/3½oz/3tbsp – 90 calories

Chunks light tuna in water – 100g/3½oz – 100 calories

Cooked chicken breast slices – 90g/3oz – 100 calories

Cooked turkey breast slices – 100g/3½oz – 100 calories

Mini falafel 2 – 50g – 100 calories

Reduced-fat hummus – 50g/1¾oz – 120 calories

Pre-cooked chicken breast – 1 – 90g/3oz – 90 calories

READ A FLAT BELLY
SUCCESS
STORY

‘

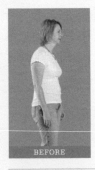

BEFORE

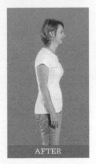

AFTER

Julie
Plavsic

AGE: 42

POUNDS LOST:

6

IN 32 DAYS

ALL-OVER
INCHES LOST:

6.5

I HAD A BABY A COUPLE OF
YEARS AGO AND SINCE THEN –
until now, anyway – I've been struggling with 10 stubborn pounds. I was on
the lower end of what I needed to lose,
but I just couldn't get the scales to
budge. I was eating healthily . . . exercising . . . nothing seemed to be
working. Of course, I have to confess, I
didn't have the most perfect eating
habits at the time.'

Julie admits to many of the behaviours that lead to a dieter's downfall.
She was grazing on 'stuff' all day long,
she says. And she wasn't always honest
with herself about what and how much
she was eating. 'Like pasta. I was
having what I thought was a small
serving of pasta, but according to the
Flat Belly Diet, I was actually having a
double or a triple portion. Who really
measures? It looked like a small portion,
so I told myself it was fine.'

At first, looking at 1,600 calories a
day, she didn't think she could do it. But
it wasn't hard, she claims, because the
food is so filling. The MUFAs amazed
her. She tried dozens of things on the
menu in the first couple of weeks, but
in the end, she needed to simplify. With
her job as an immigration lawyer and
with a small baby, Julie needed meals
that she could create quickly. 'So I
ended up having the same thing every

morning – peanut butter on toast –
which I love. And after that, I was full
until lunch. No more
snacking all morning.'

What was hard for her,
she claims, was changing her
thinking in so many ways. 'I
knew that the diet required us to
eat things like olives and olive oil. And
even though I knew that the calories
were not that bad, it was hard at first
for me to believe that you can fight fat
by eating fat. Or that fat has to do with
other things as well. I had to get over all
those years of denying myself those
high-fat foods. It was a leap of faith.'

It was a leap she's glad she took. 'I
learned so much from this diet,' she
says. 'First of all, I learned that belly fat
can be more dangerous than the other
kinds of fat, and so with this diet, I'm
making my body healthier in addition
to making it thinner. I also learned
that what the scales say is so much
less important than how you feel. I
wanted to get to 9stone 3lb, but
I'm happy with how I look and
how my clothes fit at 9stone 6lb.'

Julie doesn't consider what
she's doing a 'diet', per se. For her,
it's more a new way of looking at
food, of making choices and using
calories wisely, a way of portioning
out what you need to put in each
meal throughout the day. 'I'm
thinking about all the overweight
friends I have,' she says. 'I'm so
excited by this diet, I can't *wait* to
get them to try it!'

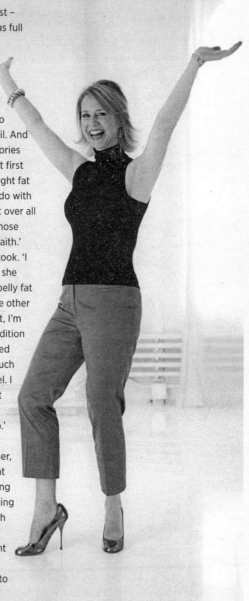

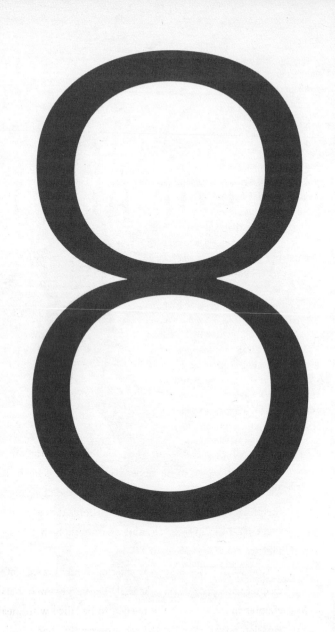

THE FOUR-WEEK PLAN: RECIPES

I HAVE A CONFESSION TO MAKE. I'm not a big cook. I have my specialities (well, speciality: canapés of mini pumpernickel bread slices spread with a melted Cheddar, olive and curry mixture) that I rely on whenever I have friends round, but for the most part, my husband's the chef in the house. He's also, bless his heart, the one who does most of the food shopping. I'm good at saying what I like (helpfully encouraging him to make things that are fresh, healthy, vegetable-filled and filling) and what would be better served when I'm away on a business trip.

Now why, you're probably wondering, would Liz start off the recipe chapter with a confession like that? Because I vowed that any recipe chapter in a book of mine needed to be filled with meals I could envision myself making. If I see a recipe that has a dozen or more ingredients and takes a day to prepare, my eyes glaze over and I start thinking about ordering a pizza.

To that end, the recipes you'll find here are sufficiently gourmet to make your mouth water and get your creative chef juices flowing. But they're also extremely simple. Take the Grilled Portobello Mushroom and Roasted Red Pepper Burgers on page 148. *It takes 4 minutes! (That's my kind of recipe!)* Or the Sweet-and-Sour Prawns on page 199 – a mere 15 minutes from start to finish. And believe me, the flavours will astound you.

But what really makes these recipes extraordinary is not how easy or fast they are to prepare but how well they fit into the *Flat Belly Diet*. Each serving contains a MUFA, for starters. As you know, MUFAs are the only foods that can specifically help reduce belly fat. You can spot them in the ingredient lists; they're in **bold**. In addition, beside most recipes is a very important component titled 'Make It a Flat Belly Diet Meal'. This box tells you what to add to one serving of that recipe to turn it into a meal that you can slot right into your menu plan. Let's say you decide to start your day with a serving of the delicious Apple Pancakes on page 142. Your MUFA is included. But remember that every meal on the *Flat Belly Diet* should equal roughly 400 calories. When you sit down to your delicious 209-calorie Apple Pancake breakfast, you should also add 240ml (8fl oz) of skimmed milk (80 calories) and 3 slices of turkey rashers (75 calories) to round out the meal and raise it to the appropriate calorie level in a healthy way. Remember, the numbers in parentheses refer to the calorie counts of specific ingredients.

Confused? Don't be. All you have to do is follow the instructions in the 'Make It a Flat Belly Diet Meal' boxes at the end of each recipe and you'll be assured of staying within the *Flat Belly Diet* rules, no matter which recipes you choose to try. Now let's get cooking.

RECIPE INDEX

SEAFOOD pp. 192–203

Steamed Salmon with Mangetout
Fish with Courgettes (Zucchini)
Roast Fish with Artichokes
Grilled Salmon Steak
Lemony Stuffed Sole
Scallop Ceviche
Chai Scallops with Pak Choi (Bok Choy)
Sweet-and-Sour Prawns
Sizzled Prawns with Tomatoes
Sesame Seared Scallops
Thai Sweet–Hot Prawns
Seared Wild Salmon with Mango Salsa

MEAT pp. 204–208

Dijon Pork Loin Chops with Cabbage
Mexican Pork Tenderloin
Stir-Fried Rice with Asian Vegetables and Beef
Vietnamese Beef Salad
Basic Balsamic Braising Steak

VEGETARIAN pp. 209–215

Broccoli and Tofu Stir-Fry with Toasted Almonds
Chickpea Salad
Courgette (Zucchini) Fusilli
Vegetable Stew
Stir-Fried Broccoli and Mushrooms with Tofu
Penne with Mushrooms and Artichokes
Soya Beans with Sesame and Spring Onions

SIDE DISHES pp. 216–222

Balsamic Roasted Carrots
Brown Rice Pilaf with Mushrooms
Courgette (Zucchini) Sauté
Wild Rice with Almond and Cranberry Dressing
Guilt-Free Chips
Stir-Fried Asparagus with Ginger, Sesame and Soya
Tuscan White Bean Spread

DESSERTS pp. 223–229

Plum and Nectarine Trifle
Chocolate Strawberries
Irresistible Brownies
Oat Cookies with Cranberries and Chocolate Chips
Chocolate Pudding with Bananas and Digestive Biscuits
Cherry–Pear Strudel
The Best-for-Last Chocolate Mousse

Frittata with Smoked Salmon and Spring Onions

Preparation time: 10 minutes / Cooking time: 15 minutes / Makes 6 servings

2tsp extra virgin olive oil

6 spring onions (whites and 2.5cm/1in of green), trimmed and coarsely chopped

6 egg whites

4 eggs

1½tsp chopped fresh tarragon or ½tsp dried

60ml (2fl oz) cold water

½tsp salt

Freshly ground black pepper

60g (2oz) thinly sliced smoked salmon, cut into 1.25cm (½in)-wide pieces

MUFA: 200g (7oz) black olive tapenade

1. Preheat the oven to 180°C/350°F/gas 4. Heat a heavy 20cm (8in) ovenproof frying pan over medium heat for 1 minute. Add the olive oil and spring onions and sauté, stirring, until soft.

2. In a medium bowl, whisk together the egg whites, eggs, tarragon, water and salt. Season with pepper. Pour the mixture into the pan and lay salmon pieces on top. Cook, stirring periodically, for about 2 minutes or until partially set.

3. Transfer to the oven and roast for about 6 to 8 minutes or until firm, golden and puffed. Remove. Use a spatula to release the frittata from the pan. Gently slide the frittata onto a warm serving platter. Spread 2 tablespoons of the tapenade on each plate, and place a slice of frittata on top.

■ **Eat One Serving:**

190

CALORIES,

10g protein, 2g carbohydrates, 15g fat, 2.5g saturated fat, 143mg cholesterol, 537mg sodium, 0g fibre

MAKE IT A FLAT BELLY DIET MEAL

Serve with 75g (2½oz) frozen dark cherries, thawed (45), mixed into 230g (8oz) fat-free plain Greek yogurt (112) and topped with 2tbsp toasted oats (37)

■ **TOTAL MEAL:**

384

CALORIES

Apple Pancakes

Preparation time: 20 minutes / Cooking time: 4 minutes / Makes 12 servings

90g (3oz) wholemeal flour

90g (3oz) unbleached plain flour

45g (1½oz) fine polenta

1tbsp baking powder

1tsp ground ginger

½tsp bicarbonate of soda

450g (1lb) fat-free plain yogurt

180ml (6fl oz) very low-fat egg substitute

2tbsp rapeseed (canola) oil

1 apple, peeled, cored and coarsely grated

MUFA: 180g (6¼oz) pecans, chopped

1. In a large bowl, mix the flours, polenta, baking powder, ginger, bicarbonate of soda, yogurt, egg substitute and oil until combined.

2. Fold the grated apples into the batter.

3. Coat a large non-stick frying pan with non-stick cooking spray and heat over medium heat.

4. For each pancake, spoon 2 to 3 tablespoons of the batter into the frying pan. Cook for 2 minutes or until bubbles appear on the surface and edges set. Flip to the other side.

5. Cook until lightly browned, about 2 minutes. Repeat with the remaining batter.

6. Top each serving with 2 tablespoons of the chopped pecans.

■ **Eat One Serving:**

209

CALORIES,

6g protein, 19g carbohydrates, 13.5g fat, 1g saturated fat, 1mg cholesterol, 208mg sodium, 3g fibre

MAKE IT A FLAT BELLY DIET MEAL

Serve with 240ml (8fl oz) skimmed milk (80) and 3 turkey rashers (75)

■ **Total Meal:**

364

CALORIES

Nutty Fruit Muffins

Preparation time: 10 minutes / Cooking time: 20 minutes / Makes 12 servings

250g (9oz) wholemeal plain flour

1½tsp baking powder

1½tsp ground cinnamon

½tsp bicarbonate of soda

¼tsp salt

230g (8oz) fat-free vanilla yogurt

90g (3oz) brown sugar

1 egg

2tbsp rapeseed (canola) oil

1tsp vanilla extract

MUFA: 180g (6¼oz) walnuts, chopped

115g (4oz) tinned crushed pineapple in juice, drained

90g (3oz) currants or raisins

30g (1oz) grated carrots

1. Preheat the oven to 200°C/400°F/gas 6.

2. In a large bowl, combine first five ingredients. In a medium bowl, combine the yogurt, brown sugar, egg, oil and vanilla extract. Stir the yogurt mixture into the flour mixture just until blended. (Lumps are OK.) Fold in the walnuts, pineapple, currants or raisins and carrots.

3. Divide the batter evenly among 12 muffin cases in a muffin tin coated with non-stick cooking spray.

4. Bake for 20 minutes or until a skewer inserted in the centre of a muffin comes out clean.

5. Cool in tin on a wire rack for 5 minutes. Remove muffins from the pan to cool completely on the wire rack.

■ **Eat One Serving:**

242

CALORIES,

6g protein, 29g carbohydrates, 12.5g fat, 1g saturated fat, 18mg cholesterol, 177mg sodium, 3g fibre

MAKE IT A FLAT BELLY DIET MEAL

Serve with 230g (8oz) fat-free plain Greek yogurt (112)

■ **Total Meal:**

354

CALORIES

Granola

Preparation and Cooking time: 45 minutes / Makes 10 servings (90g/3oz) each

230g (8oz) oatmeal

**MUFA: 150g (5½oz)
  walnuts, chopped**

75g (2½oz)
  unprocessed bran
45g (1½oz) ground
  linseed (flaxseed)
75ml (2½fl oz) apple
  juice
120ml (4fl oz) maple
  syrup
1tsp minced
  crystallized ginger
145g (5oz) dried
  apples, chopped
45g (1½oz) dried
  sweetened
  cranberries

1. Preheat the oven to 150°C/300°F/gas 2. Coat a rimmed baking sheet with cooking spray. Combine the oatmeal, walnuts, bran and linseed in a large bowl.

2. Combine the juice, syrup and ginger in a small saucepan. Cook over medium heat until the mixture simmers. Pour over the oats, stirring to coat.

3. Spread onto the prepared baking sheet. Bake for 25 to 35 minutes or until lightly browned, stirring twice. Place in a bowl and stir in the apples and cranberries.

■ **Eat One Serving:**

294

CALORIES,

7g protein, 43g carbohydrates, 12g fat, 1g saturated fat, 0mg cholesterol, 112mg sodium, 8g fibre

MAKE IT A FLAT BELLY DIET MEAL
Serve with 240ml (8fl oz) skimmed milk (118)

■ **Total Meal:**

412

CALORIES

Granola Parfait

Preparation time: 5 minutes / Makes 2 servings

1 banana, sliced
145g (5oz) raspberries
145g (5oz) fat-free
    Greek-style yogurt
230g (8oz) granola
    (home-made – see
    p.144 – or shop-
    bought)

MUFA: walnuts

1. Layer the banana, raspberries, yogurt and granola in 2 tall glasses. Serve immediately.

■ **Eat One Serving:**

420

CALORIES,
14g protein, 67g carbohydrates, 13g fat, 1g saturated fat, 0mg cholesterol, 140mg sodium, 14g fibre

A SINGLE SERVING OF THIS RECIPE COUNTS AS A FLAT BELLY DIET MEAL WITHOUT ANY ADD-ONS!

Mango Surprise Smoothie

Preparation time: 5 minutes / Makes 1 serving

30g (1oz) mango
   cubes

**MUFA: 60g (2oz)
   mashed ripe
   avocado**

120ml (4fl oz) mango
   juice
60g (2oz) fat-free
   vanilla yogurt
1tbsp freshly squeezed
   lime juice
1tbsp sugar
6 ice cubes

1. Combine the mango, avocado, lime juice, sugar and ice cubes in a blender. Process until smooth. Pour into a tall glass. Garnish with sliced mango or strawberry, if desired, and serve.

■ **Eat One Serving:**

268

CALORIES,
5g protein, 53g carbohydrates, 6g fat, 1g saturated fat, 1mg cholesterol, 84mg sodium, 4g fibre

**MAKE IT A FLAT
BELLY DIET MEAL**
Serve with 1 pear (sliced) (104)

■ **TOTAL MEAL:**

372

CALORIES

Eggs Florentine with Sun-Dried Tomato Pesto

Preparation and Cooking time: 20 minutes / Makes 4 servings

1tsp olive oil
1 packet (250g/9oz)
    pre-washed
    spinach
90g (3oz) fat-free
    Greek-style
    yogurt

MUFA: 4tbsp sun-dried tomato pesto

1tsp vinegar
Pinch of salt
4 large eggs
2 whole grain
    English muffins,
    split and toasted
Freshly ground black
    pepper

1. Heat the oil in a large non-stick frying pan over medium–high heat. Add the spinach and cook (in batches if necessary) until wilted.

2. Combine the yogurt and pesto. Stir 60g (2oz) into the spinach and remove from the heat. Cover to keep warm.

3. Meanwhile, heat a medium saucepan containing 2.5cm (1in) of water to the boil over high heat. Add the vinegar and salt and reduce the heat to low. Break an egg into a cup and gently tip the egg into the water. Repeat with the remaining 3 eggs. Cover and simmer, shaking the pan 2 or 3 times, for 3 to 5 minutes for a soft-cooked yolk or until the whites are completely set and the yolks begin to thicken.

4. Place an English muffin half on each of 4 warm plates. Divide the spinach between the muffins. Remove the eggs with a slotted spoon, and drain over paper towels (still in the spoon), before placing on the spinach.

5. Stir 1 tablespoon of the poaching liquid into the yogurt mixture to make it smoother. Spoon evenly over each egg and grind some pepper over the top.

■ Eat One Serving:

175

CALORIES,

12g protein, 21g carbohydrates, 6g fat, 2g saturated fat, 212mg cholesterol, 462mg sodium, 5g fibre

MAKE IT A FLAT BELLY DIET MEAL

Serve with 2 slices lean back bacon, grilled (140)

■ TOTAL MEAL:

315

CALORIES

Grilled Portobello Mushroom and Roasted Pepper Burgers

Preparation time: 4 minutes / Cooking time: 6 minutes / Makes 2 servings

4 small portobello
   mushrooms
   (230g/8oz total),
   stems removed
4tsp balsamic vinegar
2 roasted red pepper
   halves, from a jar
2 wholemeal burger
   buns

**MUFA: 2tbsp ready-
   prepared pesto**

4 leaves frisée
   lettuce

1. Preheat grill to medium.

2. Grill the mushrooms for 8 minutes, turning halfway during cooking and brushing with the vinegar. Warm the pepper halves and buns under the grill.

3. Spread 1 tablespoon pesto on each bun bottom, then place 2 mushrooms and 1 pepper slice on each burger bun bottom, adding 2 pieces of frisée to each. Drizzle with additional vinegar, if desired, and cap with burger bun top.

■ **Eat One Serving:**

270

CALORIES,
10g protein, 37g carbohydrates, 9.5g fat, 2.5g saturated fat, 5mg cholesterol, 614mg sodium, 5g fibre

MAKE IT A FLAT BELLY DIET MEAL
Add a dessert: mix 60g (2oz) fat-free plain yogurt (50) with 1tsp honey (21) and top with 115g (4oz) pear slices (50)

■ **TOTAL MEAL:**

391

CALORIES

Wasabi Salmon Sandwiches

Preparation time: 8 minutes / Makes 4 servings

4tbsp extra-light
    mayonnaise
1/4-1/2tsp wasabi paste
230g (8oz) tinned wild
    red salmon
8 thin slices
    wholemeal
    bread, toasted
4 thin slices red onion
4 thin slices red
    pepper

**MUFA: 1 medium
    sliced avocado**

4tbsp sliced pickled
    ginger
60g (2oz) rocket
    leaves

1. In a small bowl, combine the mayonnaise and wasabi paste until smooth. Start with 1/4 teaspoon of the paste and add more to suit your taste. Gently fold in the salmon.

2. Place 4 slices of the bread on a flat surface and top each with a quarter of the salmon mixture, 1 onion slice separated into rings, 1 pepper slice, a quarter of the avocado, 1 tablespoon ginger, and a quarter of the rocket. Top with the remaining 4 slices of bread.

■ **Eat One Serving:**

243

CALORIES,
12g protein, 26g carbohydrates, 10g fat, 1.5g saturated fat, 21mg cholesterol, 355mg sodium, 6g fibre

**MAKE IT A FLAT
BELLY DIET MEAL**
Serve with 100g (3 1/2 oz) frozen, thawed edamame (soya beans) (130)

■ **TOTAL MEAL:**

373

CALORIES

Tuna Bruschetta

Preparation time: 5 minutes / Makes 2 servings

170g (6oz) tinned
   reduced-salt
   water-packed
   tuna, drained and
   flaked
230g (8oz) tinned
   chopped
   tomatoes, drained
30g (1oz) crumbled
   reduced-fat feta
   cheese, if available

**MUFA: 4tbsp black
   olive tapenade**

1tbsp lemon juice
   4 slices wholemeal
   bread, toasted

1. In a bowl, combine the tuna, tomatoes, feta and lemon juice.

2. Spread the tapenade over 2 slices of the toast and top each with half of the tuna mixture. Top with the remaining 2 slices of toast.

■ **Eat One Serving:**

391

CALORIES,

35g protein, 30g carbohydrates, 14.5g fat, 2.5g saturated fat, 43mg cholesterol, 717mg sodium, 6g fibre

A SINGLE SERVING OF THIS RECIPE COUNTS AS A FLAT BELLY DIET MEAL WITHOUT ANY ADD-ONS!

Fresh Pea Soup with Mint

Preparation time: 7 minutes / Cooking time: 15 minutes
Chilling time: 1 hour / Makes 4 servings

1tbsp olive oil

2 spring onions, green parts only, cut into 10cm (4in) pieces

1 stick celery, trimmed and cut into 5cm (2in) pieces

½ medium onion, finely chopped

700ml (24fl oz) low-sodium chicken or vegetable stock

560g (1lb 4oz) peas, fresh or frozen and thawed

¼tsp salt

5tbsp fresh mint leaves

115g (4oz) fat-free plain Greek yogurt

MUFA: 60g (2oz) pumpkin seeds, toasted

1. Heat the oil in a large saucepan over medium–high heat. Add the spring onions, celery and onion. Cook, stirring, for about 5 minutes or until the vegetables are tender.

2. Add the stock and bring to the boil. Add the peas and salt. Simmer for 10 minutes.

3. Carefully transfer the mixture to the bowl of a food processor fitted with a metal blade or into a blender (in batches, if necessary). Add the mint. Purée until smooth. Cover and chill for at least 1 hour.

4. Spoon the soup into 4 serving bowls. Dollop 2 tablespoons of yogurt in the centre of each and sprinkle with 2 tablespoons of the pumpkin seeds.

■ **Eat One Serving:**

337

CALORIES,

23g protein, 29g carbohydrates, 16.5g fat, 3g saturated fat, 4mg cholesterol, 439mg sodium, 8g fibre

MAKE IT A FLAT BELLY DIET MEAL

Serve with 115g (4oz) grapes (60)

■ **TOTAL MEAL:**

397

CALORIES

Asian Soup with Prawn Dumplings

Preparation time: 15 minutes / Cooking time: 15 minutes / Makes 4 servings

4 cloves garlic, smashed, divided

1cm (½in) piece fresh ginger, peeled and smashed, divided

230g (8oz) medium prawns, peeled and deveined

4tbsp fresh coriander

2tsp cornflour

2tbsp water

1tbsp reduced-sodium soy sauce

½tsp toasted sesame oil

1.5l (2½ pints) low-sodium chicken stock

1 stalk lemongrass, cut in half and smashed

½tsp chilli flakes

230g (8oz) cooked kale

MUFA: 60g (2oz) dry-roasted peanuts, chopped

1. In a food processor, mince half of the garlic and ginger. Add the prawns and coriander; pulse to combine. In a small bowl, whisk together the cornflour and water until the cornflour is dissolved. Add to the food processor along with the soy sauce and oil. Pulse to combine. Set aside.

2. In a large saucepan over high heat, bring to the boil the stock, lemongrass, chilli flakes, and the remaining garlic and ginger. Reduce the heat to low and let it simmer.

3. Meanwhile, moisten your clean hands and roll the prawn mixture into 12 balls. Drop the prawn dumplings one at a time into the simmering soup. Cook for 6 minutes or until opaque. Remove and discard the lemongrass. Divide the greens evenly among 4 serving bowls and ladle the soup and 3 dumplings on top of each. Sprinkle with 2 tablespoons of the peanuts.

■ **Eat One Serving:**

252

CALORIES,
24g protein, 13g carbohydrates, 13g fat, 2g saturated fat, 86mg cholesterol, 335mg sodium, 2g fibre

MAKE IT A FLAT BELLY DIET MEAL
Serve with 150g (5½oz) red pepper slices (40) and 4tbsp hummus for dipping (100)

■ **TOTAL MEAL:**

392

CALORIES

Mexican Chicken Soup

Preparation time: 4 minutes / Cooking time: 16 minutes / Makes 4 servings

1.2l (2 pints) low-sodium chicken stock

5 corn tortillas (15cm/6in) sliced into 5mm (¼in) strips

340g (12oz) boneless, skinless chicken breast, thinly sliced crossways

2tbsp hot salsa

90g (3oz) halved cherry tomatoes

MUFA: 1 medium avocado, chopped

15g (½oz) fresh coriander leaves

1. In a large heavy saucepan, bring the stock to the boil, covered over high heat.

2. Meanwhile, scatter the tortilla strips on the grill pan. Toast, turning the strips occasionally, until golden-brown in spots, about 5 minutes. Remove the tray from the grill and set the tortilla strips aside.

3. When the stock boils, add the chicken, chilli pepper and tomatoes and return to the boil. Remove from the heat. Divide the tortilla strips, avocado and coriander leaves evenly among 4 bowls, making a mound in the centre. Ladle the soup into bowls.

■ **Eat One Serving:**

282

CALORIES,

29g protein, 24g carbohydrates, 9.5g fat, 1.5g saturated fat, 49mg cholesterol, 153mg sodium, 5g fibre

MAKE IT A FLAT BELLY DIET MEAL

Serve with 150g (5½oz) salad leaves (10) tossed with 2tbsp balsamic vinaigrette (45) and 115g (4oz) of grapes (60)

■ **TOTAL MEAL:**

397

CALORIES

Slow Cooker Chilli

Preparation time: 10 minutes / Cooking time: 4 to 6 hours / Makes 4 servings

2 x 400g (14oz) tins whole tomatoes
1 medium green pepper, seeded and chopped
1 x tin 420g (14½oz) kidney beans, rinsed and drained
340g (12oz) fat-free soya mince
Chilli powder
1tbsp onion, finely chopped
1tbsp olive oil

MUFA: 1 medium avocado, chopped

1. In a slow cooker, combine the tomatoes, pepper, beans, soya mince, chilli powder to taste, onion and oil. Cover and cook on high setting for 4 to 6 hours or on medium setting for 8 hours or until thickened. Garnish each serving with ¼ of the avocado.

■ **Eat One Serving:**

358

CALORIES,
24g protein,
34g carbohydrates,
13.5g fat, 2g saturated fat, 0mg cholesterol, 807mg sodium, 13g fibre

A SINGLE SERVING OF THIS RECIPE COUNTS AS A FLAT BELLY DIET MEAL WITHOUT ANY ADD-ONS!

Black Bean Chilli

Preparation time: 5 minutes / Cooking time: 3 minutes / Makes 2 servings

230g (8oz) fat-free
soya mince
1 x tin 420g (14½oz)
no-salt-added
black beans, rinsed
and drained
230g (8oz) crushed
tomato salsa with
chilli, garlic and
lime
2tsp chilli powder
1tsp ground cumin

**MUFA: ½ a medium
avocado, mashed**

1. In a saucepan over medium heat, combine the soya mince, beans, salsa, chilli powder and cumin. Cook, stirring occasionally, for about 3 minutes or until heated through. Top each serving with half the mashed avocado.

■ **Eat One Serving:**

338

CALORIES,
20g protein, 39g
carbohydrates,
9g fat, 1.7g
saturated fat, 0mg
cholesterol, 674mg
sodium, 15g fibre

**MAKE IT A FLAT
BELLY DIET MEAL**
Serve with 150g
(5½oz) sliced red
pepper (40)

■ **TOTAL MEAL:**

378

CALORIES

Hearty Country Vegetable Soup

Preparation time: 15 minutes / Cooking time: 2 hours 15 minutes
Makes 8 servings

**MUFA: 120ml (4fl oz)
olive oil, divided**

½ large onion,
chopped
3 sticks celery,
chopped
1 small head green
cabbage, chopped
2 carrots, chopped
2 cloves garlic, finely
chopped
115g (4oz) dried white
beans
1.2l (2 pints) low-
sodium vegetable
stock
1½tsp chopped fresh
thyme or ½tsp
dried
1½tsp chopped fresh
savory or sage or
½tsp dried
230g (8oz) green
beans, cut into
2.5cm (1in) pieces
1 courgette (zucchini),
halved lengthways
and sliced

1. Heat 4 tablespoons oil in a
large pan over medium–low
heat. Stir in the onion, celery,
cabbage, carrots and garlic.
Cover and cook for 12 to 15
minutes, stirring occasionally.
Add the beans and 1l (1¾
pints) of the stock. Bring the
mixture to the boil. Reduce the
heat to medium–low and stir in
the thyme and savory. Cover
and cook for 1 to 1½ hours or
until the beans are almost
tender, adding some of the
remaining stock if the soup
becomes too thick.

2. Stir in the green beans and
courgette (zucchini). Partially
cover and cook for 20 to 30
minutes or until the green
beans are tender. Divide
among 8 bowls. Drizzle ½
tablespoon of the remaining oil
in each bowl.

■ **Eat One Serving:**

237

CALORIES,
6g protein, 23g
carbohydrates, 14g
fat, 2g saturated
fat, 0mg
cholesterol, 353mg
sodium, 7g fibre

**MAKE IT A FLAT
BELLY DIET MEAL**
Serve with 115g
(4oz) baby salad
leaves (15) and 115g
(4oz) halved cherry
tomatoes (30)
tossed with 2tbsp
fat-free salad
dressing (90)

■ **TOTAL MEAL:**

372

CALORIES

Turnip and Carrot Soup with Parmesan

Preparation time: 15 minutes / Cooking time: 20 minutes / Makes 8 servings

450g (1lb) white turnips, peeled and quartered

4 large carrots, cut into chunks

2 large red or white new potatoes, quartered

1 large onion, chopped

5 cloves garlic, smashed

350ml (12fl oz) low-sodium chicken stock

350ml (12fl oz) water

1½tsp chopped fresh thyme or ½tsp dried

1½tsp chopped fresh sage or ½tsp dried

¼tsp salt

¼tsp freshly ground black pepper

240ml (8fl oz) skimmed milk

60g (2oz) grated Parmesan cheese

MUFA: 120g (4¼oz) pine nuts, toasted

1. In a large saucepan, combine the turnips, carrots, potatoes, onion, garlic, stock, water, thyme, sage, salt and pepper. Bring to the boil over high heat. Reduce the heat to medium, cover and simmer for 20 minutes or until the vegetables are very tender.

2. In batches, transfer the cooked vegetables into the bowl of a food processor fitted with a metal blade or into a blender, and purée until smooth. When all the soup has been puréed, return it to the pan. Stir in the milk. Cook over low heat just until heated through (do not boil). Remove from the heat and stir in the Parmesan. Ladle into bowls and top each with 2 tablespoons of pine nuts.

■ **Eat One Serving:**

261

CALORIES,

9g protein, 28g carbohydrates, 13.5g fat, 2g saturated fat, 7mg cholesterol, 263mg sodium, 5g fibre

MAKE IT A FLAT BELLY DIET MEAL

Serve with 2 Laughing Cow® Light Cheese wedges (70) and 2 Ryvita® crispbreads (64)

■ **TOTAL MEAL:**

394

CALORIES

Creamy Broccoli Soup

Preparation and cooking time: 35 minutes / Makes 4 servings

MUFA: 4tbsp (60ml) olive oil, divided

1 onion, chopped
960ml (32fl oz) low-sodium vegetable stock
450g (1lb) broccoli crowns, chopped
115g (4oz) fresh spinach
5tbsp plain flour
½ tsp salt
¼ tsp freshly grated nutmeg
Freshly ground black pepper

1. Heat 1 tablespoon of the oil in a large pot over medium-high heat. Add the onion and cook, stirring occasionally, for 8 minutes or until golden brown.

2. Add the stock and broccoli. Cover, reduce the heat to low and simmer for 15 minutes or until the broccoli is tender. Turn off the heat, add the spinach and stir until the spinach is wilted. Transfer the mixture to a blender or leave it in the pot if using a hand-held blender. Purée until smooth.

3. Meanwhile, heat the remaining 3 tablespoons oil in a small pan over medium heat. Add the flour and stir until smooth. Cook, stirring occasionally, for 2 to 3 minutes or until light brown. Set aside.

4. Heat the soup in a pot over medium-high heat just until it begins to boil. Reduce the heat to low to maintain a simmer. Add the reserved flour mixture and stir until the soup thickens.

5. Add the salt, nutmeg and pepper to taste.

■ **Eat One Serving:**

200
CALORIES,

6g protein, 17g carbohydrates, 14g fat, 2g saturated fat, 0mg cholesterol, 480mg sodium, 6g fibre

MAKE IT A FLAT BELLY DIET MEAL
Serve with 5 Ryvita® Rye crispbreads (160)

■ **TOTAL MEAL:**

360
CALORIES

Cucumber and Melon Salad with Watercress, Herbs and Feta

Preparation time: 25 minutes / Makes 4 servings

DRESSING
2tsp extra virgin olive oil
2tbsp freshly squeezed lemon juice
2tbsp white wine vinegar
1tbsp finely chopped shallot
1tsp sugar
$\frac{1}{2}$tsp salt
$\frac{1}{2}$tsp freshly ground black pepper

SALAD
3 cucumbers, peeled and chopped
1 honeydew melon, or other type, scooped into balls
1 bunch watercress, large stems discarded
30g (1oz) fresh mint leaves
60g (2oz) crumbled feta cheese

MUFA: 60g (2oz) pine nuts, toasted

1tbsp chopped kalamata olives

1. To prepare the dressing: in a small bowl, whisk together the oil, lemon juice, vinegar, shallot, sugar, salt and pepper.

2. To prepare the salad: in a large bowl, combine the cucumbers, melon balls, watercress, mint, feta, pine nuts and olives. Pour the dressing on the salad and toss gently to coat.

■ **Eat One Serving:**

354

CALORIES,
9g protein, 43g carbohydrates, 19g fat, 4g saturated fat, 17mg cholesterol, 548mg sodium, 5g fibre

A SINGLE SERVING OF THIS RECIPE COUNTS AS A FLAT BELLY DIET MEAL WITHOUT ANY ADD-ONS!

Carrot–Walnut Salad

Preparation time: 20 minutes / Makes 4 servings

90g (3oz) golden
    raisins
2tbsp rice wine
    vinegar
1tbsp rapeseed
    (canola) oil
2tsp freshly squeezed
    lemon juice (about
    1 lemon)
1tsp honey
⅛tsp salt
4 large carrots, grated

MUFA: 60g (2oz) walnuts, toasted and chopped

15g (½oz) chopped
    fresh Italian
    parsley

1. Soak the raisins in hot water for 20 minutes to plump them. Drain.

2. In a small bowl, whisk together the vinegar, oil, lemon juice, honey and salt to make a dressing.

3. Combine the carrots, walnuts, parsley, raisins and dressing in a medium bowl and toss to coat. Divide evenly among 4 salad plates.

■ **Eat One Serving:**

199

CALORIES,

3g protein, 20g carbohydrates, 13.5g fat, 1.5g saturated fat, 0mg cholesterol, 127mg sodium, 4 g fibre

MAKE IT A FLAT BELLY DIET MEAL

Serve with 1 slice rye bread (80) and 1 apple (80)

■ **TOTAL MEAL:**

359

CALORIES

Sugar Snap Pea and Fennel Salad with Apple Cider Vinaigrette

Preparation time: 15 minutes / Makes 6 servings

2tbsp apple cider
vinegar
2tsp honey
1½tsp extra virgin
olive oil
¾tsp Dijon mustard
¼tsp salt
300g (10½oz) sugar
snap peas, tough
strings removed
300g (10½oz) shelled
fresh peas
1 small fennel bulb,
trimmed, halved
and cut into
bite-sized strips
¼ mild onion, grated
1tbsp chopped fresh
tarragon
2tsp finely chopped
shallots
Freshly ground black
pepper

MUFA: 90g (3oz)
sunflower seeds

1. Whisk together the vinegar, honey, oil, mustard and salt in a large bowl. Add the sugar snap peas, peas, fennel, onion, tarragon and shallot. Toss to coat and season to taste with pepper. Divide evenly among 6 salad plates and sprinkle with the sunflower seeds.

■ **Eat One Serving:**

189

CALORIES,

8g protein, 19g
carbohydrates,
10.5g fat, 1g
saturated fat, 0mg
cholesterol, 141mg
sodium, 6g fibre

MAKE IT A FLAT
BELLY DIET MEAL
Serve with 60g
(2oz) tinned wild
red salmon (180)

■ **TOTAL MEAL:**

369

CALORIES

Crab Salad with Avocado and Grapefruit

Preparation time: 22 minutes / Makes 4 servings

DRESSING

2 tbsp orange juice

2 tsp extra virgin olive oil

2 tbsp white wine vinegar

2 tsp finely chopped fresh tarragon or chervil

1/2 tsp freshly grated orange zest

1/2 tsp salt

1/4 tsp mustard powder

1/4 tsp freshly ground black pepper

SALAD

2 heads butterhead lettuce, separated into leaves

2 medium mild onions, sliced

2 grapefruit, peeled and cut into sections (see Note)

MUFA: 1 medium avocado, sliced

230g (8oz) white crabmeat

1 tbsp chopped blanched hazelnuts, toasted

1. To prepare the dressing: in a medium bowl, whisk together the orange juice, oil, vinegar, tarragon or chervil, orange zest, salt, mustard and pepper.

2. To prepare the salad: in a large bowl, combine the lettuce, onions and grapefruit. Add the dressing and toss to coat. Arrange the salad evenly among 4 plates. Top with avocado slices, 1/4 of the crabmeat and hazelnuts.

Note: Replace the grapefruit with pomelos if you can find them.

▨ Eat One Serving:

237
CALORIES,
11g protein, 31g carbohydrates, 10g fat, 1.5g saturated fat, 30mg cholesterol, 335mg sodium, 7g fibre

MAKE IT A FLAT BELLY DIET MEAL

Serve with 4 Ryvita® crispbreads (128)

▨ TOTAL MEAL:

365
CALORIES

Curried Pearl Barley and Prawn Salad

Preparation time: 20 minutes / Cooking time: 45 minutes / Makes 6 servings

700ml (1¼ pints) water

1tsp curry powder

½tsp turmeric

230g (8oz) pearl barley

5tbsp freshly squeezed lime juice (about 4 limes)

1tbsp vegetable oil

2tsp finely chopped jalapeño chilli pepper, seeded (see Note)

1 clove garlic, finely chopped

¼tsp salt

450g (1lb) small cooked prawns, peeled and deveined

450g (1lb) seeded and diced tomatoes

1 chopped green pepper

⅓ cucumber, chopped and peeled

800g (1lb 12oz) baby salad leaves

4tbsp chopped fresh basil

MUFA: 90g (3oz) pumpkin seeds, toasted

1. In a large saucepan over high heat, bring the water, curry powder and turmeric to the boil. Stir in the pearl barley. Cover and reduce the heat to low. Cook for about 45 minutes or until the water is absorbed and the barley is tender. Remove from heat. Meanwhile, in a large bowl, whisk together the lime juice, oil, chilli pepper, garlic and salt. Add the prawns, tomatoes, pepper, cucumber and pearl barley. Toss to coat.

2. Spoon the salad on top of a portion of baby salad leaves per plate. Divide salad evenly and sprinkle with the basil and the pumpkin seeds.

Note: Wear plastic gloves and keep hands away from eyes when handling fresh chilli peppers.

■ **Eat One Serving:**

338

CALORIES,

24g protein, 35g carbohydrates, 12.5g fat, 2.5g saturated fat, 115mg cholesterol, 273mg sodium, 7g fibre

MAKE IT A FLAT BELLY DIET MEAL

Serve on a bed of 75g (2½oz) baby greens (15)

■ **TOTAL MEAL:**

353

CALORIES

Beetroot and Goat's Cheese Salad

Preparation time: 25 minutes / Makes 6 servings

SALAD

400g (14oz) baby
  salad leaves
8 medium tinned
  beetroot (about
  230g/8oz),
  drained and sliced

**MUFA: 90g (3oz)
toasted walnut
halves**

DRESSING

2tsp olive oil
3tbsp white wine
  vinegar
¼tsp salt
Freshly ground black
  pepper
60g (2oz) soft goat's
  cheese, crumbled

1. To prepare the salad:
combine the baby salad
leaves, beetroot and walnuts
in a large bowl.

2. To prepare the dressing:
pour the olive oil into a small
bowl and gradually whisk in
the vinegar and salt. Season to
taste with pepper. Pour over
the salad and toss gently.
Divide evenly among 6 plates
and sprinkle with the cheese.

■ **Eat One Serving:**

147

CALORIES,

5g protein, 6g
carbohydrates,
12.5g fat, 3g
saturated fat, 7mg
cholesterol, 227 mg
sodium, 2g fibre

**MAKE IT A FLAT
BELLY DIET MEAL**

Serve with
wholemeal pitta
(140) and 4tbsp
hummus (100)

■ **TOTAL MEAL:**

387

CALORIES

Warm Quinoa Salad

Preparation time: 8 minutes / Cooking time: 10 minutes / Makes 4 servings

480ml (16fl oz) water
230g (8oz) quinoa, rinsed and drained
½ head chopped radicchio plus leaves for garnish
8tbsp chopped fresh coriander
115g (4oz) golden raisins
120ml (4fl oz) fat-free honey mustard dressing
½tsp salt
Freshly ground black pepper

MUFA: 60g (2oz) cashews, toasted and chopped

1. In a medium saucepan, over high heat, bring the water and quinoa to the boil. Reduce the heat to a simmer, cover and cook for about 5 minutes or until all the liquid is absorbed.

2. Transfer the quinoa to a medium serving bowl. Add the chopped radicchio, coriander, raisins, dressing and salt. Toss to coat. Season to taste with pepper. Place the radicchio leaves onto 4 plates, divide the salad evenly and sprinkle each with ¼ of the cashews.

■ **Eat One Serving:**

363

CALORIES,
9g protein, 60g carbohydrates, 10.5g fat, 2g saturated fat, 0mg cholesterol, 435mg sodium, 4g fibre

A SINGLE SERVING OF THIS RECIPE COUNTS AS A FLAT BELLY DIET MEAL WITHOUT ANY ADD-ONS!

Italian Prawn and Pasta Salad

Preparation time: 7 minutes / Cooking time: 10 minutes / Makes 2 servings

115g (4oz) wholemeal
fusilli pasta
90g (3oz) frozen
prawns, drained
60g (2oz) halved
cherry tomatoes
4tbsp torn fresh basil
1tsp Italian herb
seasoning
1tsp olive oil

**MUFA: 30g (1oz) pine
nuts, toasted**

1. In a medium pan of rapidly boiling water, cook the pasta for 8 to 10 minutes or until al dente. Drain and rinse with cold water until cool to the touch.

2. In a large bowl, combine the prawns, tomatoes, basil, Italian herb seasoning, oil and pasta. Toss to coat and sprinkle with the nuts.

■ **Eat One Serving:**

231
CALORIES,

12g protein, 15g carbohydrates, 15g fat, 1g saturated fat, 87mg cholesterol, 362mg sodium, 3g fibre

MAKE IT A FLAT BELLY DIET MEAL
Serve with 1 cheese string (80) and 115g (4oz) grapes (60)

■ **TOTAL MEAL:**

371
CALORIES

Turkey–Avocado Salad

Preparation time: 8 minutes / Cooking time: 7 minutes / Makes 4 servings

450g (1lb) turkey
    breast fillets
2tsp olive oil, plus 1tsp
    for the turkey
2tbsp cider vinegar
1tbsp water
1tsp Dijon mustard
500g (1lb 2oz) baby
    spinach
4 cooked turkey
    rashers, chopped

**MUFA: 1 medium
    avocado, diced**

4 cherry tomatoes,
    halved
30g (1oz) blue cheese,
    crumbled
Freshly ground black
    pepper

1. Preheat the grill on medium–high heat for 2 minutes. Brush the turkey with 1 teaspoon of the oil. Grill the turkey for 4 minutes, turn over and continue cooking for about 3 minutes more or until no longer pink. Cut into chunks.

2. In a jar, combine the vinegar, water, mustard and the remaining 2 teaspoons oil. Cover and shake well.

3. In a large bowl, combine the spinach with 2 tablespoons of the dressing. Toss to coat the leaves. Arrange the turkey, cooked turkey rashers, avocados, tomatoes and cheese over the spinach. Drizzle on the remaining dressing, and season with pepper to taste.

■ **Eat One Serving:**

288

CALORIES,
34g protein, 10g carbohydrates, 13.5g fat, 3.1g saturated fat, 57mg cholesterol, 473mg sodium, 5g fibre

MAKE IT A FLAT BELLY DIET MEAL
Serve with 1 medium apple (80)

■ **TOTAL MEAL:**

368

CALORIES

Soba Noodle Salad with Mangetout

Preparation time: 15 minutes / Makes 6 servings

230g (8oz) dry soba noodles or wholewheat spaghetti

2tbsp honey

2tbsp freshly squeezed lime juice (about 2 limes)

2tbsp rice wine vinegar

2tbsp reduced-sodium soy sauce

1tbsp grated fresh ginger

¼tsp red chilli pepper flakes

2tbsp peanut (groundnut) oil

450g (1lb) shredded cooked chicken

170g (6oz) fresh mangetout, cut in thin strips

2 red peppers, seeded and thinly sliced lengthways

115g (4oz) grated carrot

MUFA: 240g (8½oz) avocado, diced

4tbsp fresh coriander, coarsely chopped

1. Cook the noodles according to the packet directions. Drain and rinse with cold water. Set aside.

2. In a large bowl, whisk together the honey, lime juice, vinegar, soy sauce, ginger and chilli pepper flakes. Whisk in the oil in a steady stream.

3. Fold in the chicken, mangetout, peppers, carrots, avocado, coriander and noodles.

■ **Eat One Serving:**

352

CALORIES,

20g protein, 48g carbohydrates, 11g fat, 2g saturated fat, 26mg cholesterol, 392mg sodium, 6g fibre

A SINGLE SERVING OF THIS RECIPE COUNTS AS A FLAT BELLY DIET MEAL WITHOUT ANY ADD-ONS!

Spinach Salad

Preparation time: 8 minutes / Makes 1 serving

2tbsp balsamic
  vinegar

**MUFA: 1tbsp
  olive oil**

pinch freshly ground
  black pepper
170g (6oz) fresh baby
  spinach leaves
60g (2oz) sliced
  mushrooms
30g (1oz) halved
  yellow cherry
  tomatoes
1 small red pepper,
  seeded and sliced
  into strips

1. In a salad or pasta bowl, whisk together the vinegar, oil and black pepper. Add the spinach and toss to coat. Top with the mushrooms, tomatoes and pepper.

■ **Eat One Serving:**

209

CALORIES,

4g protein, 20g carbohydrates, 14g fat, 2g saturated fat, 0mg cholesterol, 353mg sodium, 6g fibre

MAKE IT A FLAT BELLY DIET MEAL

Serve with 4 Ryvita® crispbreads (128) and 2 Laughing Cow® Light wedges (70)

■ **TOTAL MEAL:**

407

CALORIES

Herb and Mesclun Salad with Grilled Prawns

Preparation time: 30 minutes / Marinating time: 20 minutes
Cooking time: 4 minutes / Makes 4 servings

60ml (2fl oz) fresh
lime juice, divided
(about 4 limes)
½tsp ground cumin,
divided
¼tsp salt, divided
¼tsp chilli flakes,
divided
450g (1lb) large
prawns, peeled
and deveined
400g (14oz) mixed
baby salad leaves
60g (2oz) fresh mint
60g (2oz) fresh
coriander
60g (2oz) fresh
flat-leaf parsley
1 small red onion,
thinly sliced
2tbsp vegetable oil

**MUFA: 60g (2oz)
slivered almonds,
toasted**

1. In medium bowl, whisk together 2 tablespoons of the lime juice, ¼ teaspoon of the cumin, ⅛ teaspoon of the salt and a pinch of the chilli flakes. Stir in the prawns and chill for 20 minutes.

2. Meanwhile, in a serving bowl, toss together the baby salad leaves, mint, coriander, parsley and onion. Chill until ready to serve.

3. In a small bowl, whisk together the oil, ¼ teaspoon cumin, ⅛ teaspoon salt, the remaining chilli flakes and 2 tablespoons of the lime juice.

4. Grill the prawns for about 2 minutes each side or until just opaque. Add the prawns and dressing to the baby salad leaves. Toss gently to coat. Divide evenly among 4 plates and top with the almonds.

■ Eat One Serving:

280

CALORIES,
25g protein, 11g carbohydrates, 16g fat, 1.5g saturated fat, 151mg cholesterol, 327mg sodium, 5g fibre

MAKE IT A FLAT BELLY DIET MEAL
Serve with ½ wholemeal pitta (70) and 2tbsp hummus (50)

■ TOTAL MEAL:

400

CALORIES

Curried Potato Salad

Preparation time: 10 minutes / Makes 4 servings

450g (1lb) potatoes,
    boiled and cubed
2 spring onions,
    chopped

**MUFA: 60g (2oz)
    sliced almonds,
    toasted**

60g (2oz) raisins
115g (4oz) fat-free
    plain yogurt
2tbsp mango chutney
2tsp curry powder

1. Place the potatoes in a large bowl and stir in the spring onions, almonds and raisins.

2. In a small bowl, whisk together the yogurt, chutney and curry powder. Pour over the potatoes and toss to combine well. Divide evenly among 4 plates and serve.

■ **Eat One Serving:**

226

CALORIES,

6g protein, 39g carbohydrates, 6.5g fat, 0.5g saturated fat, 1mg cholesterol, 26mg sodium, 4g dietary fibre

MAKE IT A FLAT BELLY DIET MEAL
Serve on a bed of 115g (4oz) baby salad leaves (15) with 90g (3oz) grilled chicken breast (90) and 1 medium apple (80)

■ **TOTAL MEAL:**

411

CALORIES

Spinach with Hot Vinaigrette Dressing

Preparation time: 5 minutes / Cooking time: 7 minutes / Makes 4 servings

8tbsp balsamic vinegar

2tsp honey

1tsp Dijon mustard

2 cloves garlic, finely chopped

1½tsp chopped fresh tarragon or ½tsp dried

⅛tsp freshly ground black pepper

230g (8oz) leaf spinach

2 turkey rashers, cooked until crisp and crumbled

MUFA: 60g (2oz) pine nuts, toasted

1. Arrange the greens on 4 salad plates.

2. In a medium saucepan, whisk together the vinegar, honey, mustard, garlic, tarragon and pepper. Cook over medium heat for 1 to 2 minutes or until the mixture is hot but not boiling.

3. Spoon immediately over the greens and toss well to coat. Sprinkle each salad evenly with bacon and pine nuts.

■ **Eat One Serving:**

198

CALORIES,

5g protein, 18g carbohydrates, 13g fat, 2g saturated fat, 8mg cholesterol, 141mg sodium, 2g fibre

MAKE IT A FLAT BELLY DIET MEAL

Serve with 90g (3oz) grilled pork tenderloin (115) and 50g (1¾oz) steamed brown rice (55)

■ **TOTAL MEAL:**

368

CALORIES

Moroccan Carrot Salad with Toasted Cumin

Preparation time: 10 minutes / Cooking time: 2 minutes / Makes 4 servings

¾tsp ground cumin

¼tsp ground coriander

115g (4oz) sour cream, reduced-fat if available

MUFA: 4tbsp organic cold-pressed flaxseed (linseed) oil

1tbsp plus 1tsp lemon juice (about 1 lemon)

1½tsp extra virgin olive oil

¼tsp freshly grated orange zest

¼tsp salt

7 medium carrots, peeled and grated

115g (4oz) currants or unsweetened raisins

2tbsp finely chopped red onion

1. In a small, dry frying pan over medium heat, toast the cumin and coriander, stirring often, for 2 minutes or until fragrant and slightly darker in colour. Place in a medium bowl and let cool. Stir in the sour cream, flaxseed (linseed) oil, lemon juice, olive oil, orange zest and salt.

2. Add the carrots, currants and onion, and toss to coat well. Divide evenly among 4 plates.

■ Eat One Serving:

276

CALORIES,

3g protein, 26g carbohydrates, 19.5g fat, 4g saturated fat, 12mg cholesterol, 234mg sodium, 4g fibre

MAKE IT A FLAT BELLY DIET MEAL

Serve with 90g (3oz) grilled medium prawns (90)

■ TOTAL MEAL:

366

CALORIES

Spinach Salad with Radishes and Walnuts

Preparation time: 10 minutes / Makes 4 servings

1tbsp freshly squeezed lemon juice (about 1 lemon)

2tsp white wine vinegar

Salt

Freshly ground black pepper

60ml (2fl oz) extra virgin olive oil

145g (5oz) baby spinach leaves

4 medium radishes, thinly sliced

MUFA: 60g (2oz) walnut halves

1. In a large bowl, whisk together the lemon juice and vinegar. Season to taste with salt and pepper. Whisk in the olive oil slowly.

2. When ready to serve, toss together the spinach and radishes and toss with the dressing to coat. Divide evenly among 4 salad plates and sprinkle each with a ¼ of the walnuts.

■ **Eat One Serving:**

224
CALORIES,

3g protein, 6g carbohydrates, 22g fat, 2.5g saturated fat, 0mg cholesterol, 204mg sodium, 3g fibre

MAKE IT A FLAT BELLY DIET MEAL

Serve with 90g (3oz) tuna chunks in water, drained (120), and 115g (4oz) grapes (60)

■ **TOTAL MEAL:**

404
CALORIES

Broccoli, Cherry Tomato and Pesto Pasta Salad

Preparation time: 35 minutes / Makes 4 servings

115g (4oz) fusilli pasta

170g (6oz) broccoli florets

90g (3oz) cherry tomatoes, halved

1/4 red onion, thinly sliced

15g (1 1/2 oz) fresh basil, thinly sliced

MUFA: 4tbsp pesto, home-made or shop-bought

2 tbsp olive oil

1. Bring a large pot of lightly salted water to the boil. Add the fusilli and cook as per the packet directions. Add the broccoli during the last 2 minutes of cooking. Drain, rinse under cold water and drain again. Transfer to a large bowl.

2. Add the tomatoes, onion and basil to the bowl with the pasta. Combine the pesto and oil in a separate bowl. Stir the pesto mixture into the pasta and toss well. Refrigerate until ready to serve.

■ **Eat One Serving:**

288

CALORIES,

8g protein, 36g carbohydrates, 13g fat, 2g saturated fat, 1mg cholesterol, 105mg sodium, 3g fibre

MAKE IT A FLAT BELLY DIET MEAL

Serve with half of the Grilled Portobello Mushroom and Roasted Red Pepper Burger, p.148 (135)

■ **TOTAL MEAL:**

423

CALORIES

Crisp Romaine Lettuce Salad with Chicken and Mango

Preparation time: 25 minutes / Cooking time: 15 minutes / Makes 4 servings

2tbsp olive oil, divided

3 boneless, skinless chicken breasts, trimmed (170g/6oz each)

1/2tsp salt, divided

1/4tsp freshly ground black pepper, divided

2 shallots, finely chopped

2tbsp balsamic vinegar, divided

115g (4oz) shredded romaine lettuce

1 small bunch watercress, large stems discarded

45g (1½oz) finely shredded red cabbage

1 firm ripe mango, stoned, peeled and cut into 1cm (½in) pieces

MUFA: 60g (2oz) pumpkin seeds, toasted

1. Heat 1 tablespoon oil in a large non-stick frying pan over medium heat. Season both sides of the chicken with 1/4 teaspoon salt and 1/8 teaspoon pepper. Cook, turning once, about 6 minutes on each side or until a thermometer inserted in the thickest portion registers 71°C (160°F). Transfer to a plate; cover and chill completely.

2. Add the shallots and 1 tablespoon vinegar to the frying pan and cook, stirring, for about 3 minutes or until the liquid is almost evaporated. Transfer to a small bowl. Whisk in the remaining 1 tablespoon oil, 1 tablespoon vinegar, 1/4 teaspoon salt and 1/8 teaspoon pepper.

3. In a serving bowl, toss together the romaine lettuce, watercress, cabbage and mango. Cut the chicken diagonally into long, thin strips. Add to the romaine mixture and toss with dressing and pumpkin seeds.

■ **Eat One Serving:**

301
CALORIES,
33g protein, 19g carbohydrates, 10.5g fat, 2g saturated fat, 74mg cholesterol, 384mg sodium, 3g fibre

MAKE IT A FLAT BELLY DIET MEAL
Serve with 3 Ryvita® crispbreads (96)

■ **TOTAL MEAL:**

397
CALORIES

Greek Lemon Chicken

Preparation time: 18 minutes / Cooking time: 45 minutes / Makes 4 servings

4 skinless, split, bone-in chicken breasts, trimmed (about 685g/1½lb)

1 medium red pepper, seeded and cut into 8 wedges

1 medium orange pepper, seeded and cut into 8 wedges

1 medium waxy potato, cut into 8 wedges

1 medium red onion, peeled and cut into 8 wedges

MUFA: 40 stoned kalamata olives, crushed

1tbsp extra virgin olive oil

Grated zest and juice of 1 lemon

1tbsp finely chopped garlic

1tbsp chopped fresh oregano or 1tsp dried

¾tsp freshly ground black pepper

¾tsp paprika

1. Preheat the oven to 200°C/400°F/gas 6. Tear off 2 sheets of non-stick aluminium foil, each 60cm (24in) long. Put dull (non-stick) sides together, and fold over the edge on one side twice to make a seam. Open up and line and cover the edges of a 40 x 30cm (17 x 12in) rimmed baking pan (the foil's dull side should face up).

2. Place the chicken on one side of the baking tin and the peppers, potatoes, onion and olives on the other. In a bowl, whisk together the oil, lemon zest and juice, garlic, oregano, salt, black pepper and paprika. Drizzle over the chicken and vegetables, and toss to coat.

3. Roast for 40 to 45 minutes, turning the chicken and vegetables halfway through cooking or until a meat thermometer registers 74°C (165°F) when inserted into the thickest part of the chicken. Arrange 1 chicken breast and ¼ of the vegetables on 4 plates.

■ **Eat One Serving:**

401

CALORIES,

39g protein, 19g carbohydrates, 18g fat, 2.5g saturated fat, 115mg cholesterol, 742mg sodium, 3g fibre

A SINGLE SERVING OF THIS RECIPE COUNTS AS A FLAT BELLY DIET MEAL WITHOUT ANY ADD-ONS!

Spinach-Stuffed Chicken Roulade

Preparation time: 8 minutes / Cooking time: 25 minutes / Makes 4 servings

45g (1½oz) finely chopped onion
1 clove garlic, finely chopped
¼tsp chilli flakes (or to taste)
2tsp olive oil, divided
1tbsp water
4tbsp freshly grated Parmesan cheese
280g (10oz) frozen chopped spinach, thawed, drained and squeezed dry
4 chicken breast fillets (about 450g/1lb)
2tbsp sun-dried tomatoes, chopped
120ml (4fl oz) low-sodium chicken stock

MUFA: 60g (2oz) pine nuts, toasted

1. In a medium non-stick frying pan over medium heat, cook the onion, garlic and chilli flakes in 1 teaspoon oil for 30 seconds. Reduce the heat to low, cover and cook, stirring once, for about 3 minutes or until softened. In a small bowl, combine the onion mixture, Parmesan and spinach.

2. Lay the chicken on a work surface, smooth side down. Sprinkle the tomatoes evenly on the chicken. Spread the spinach mixture evenly over fillets. Roll up the fillet, ending with narrow tip, and secure with wooden cocktail sticks.

3. Add the remaining oil to the frying pan set over medium heat. Add the chicken and cook for about 10 minutes. Add the stock. Cover and cook over low heat for about 7 minutes. Transfer the roulades to a serving platter. Cover to keep warm. Boil the juices in the frying pan for about 5 minutes. Cut the roulades into diagonal slices. Drizzle with the pan juices and sprinkle with nuts.

■ **Eat One Serving:**

322

CALORIES,
33g protein, 8g carbohydrates, 17g fat, 2.5g saturated fat, 70mg cholesterol, 302mg sodium, 2g fibre

MAKE IT A FLAT BELLY DIET MEAL
Serve with 1 medium orange (70)

■ **TOTAL MEAL:**

392

CALORIES

Chicken with Citrus–Avocado Salsa

Preparation time: 8 minutes / Cooking time: 15 minutes / Makes 4 servings

4 boneless, skinless
    chicken breast
    halves (about
    685g/1½lb)
1l (1¾ pints) water
½tsp plus
    ⅛tsp salt
1 ruby red grapefruit

**MUFA: 1 medium
    avocado, diced**

4 radishes, thinly
    sliced
15g (½oz) chopped
    basil leaves
Fresh basil (optional)

1. In a large saucepan, combine the chicken, water and ½tsp salt. Cover and bring to the boil over high heat. Turn off the heat and let sit for 15 minutes or until a thermometer inserted in the thickest portion registers 74°C (165°F).

2. Meanwhile, with a knife, remove the peel and pith from the grapefruit. Working over a bowl to catch the juice, free each segment from its membrane and cut the segments into bite-size pieces, dropping them into the bowl. Add the avocado, radishes, basil and the remaining ⅛ teaspoon salt. Gently toss to mix.

3. Drain the chicken breasts, discarding the liquid. Cut crossways into 1cm (½in) slices. Divide the grapefruit mixture between 4 plates and add one piece of the chicken to each, drizzling with juice from mixture. Garnish with basil leaves, if using.

■ **Eat One Serving:**

269

CALORIES,
41g protein, 9g carbohydrates, 7.5g fat, 1.5g saturated fat, 99mg cholesterol, 188mg sodium, 3g fibre

MAKE IT A FLAT BELLY DIET MEAL
Serve with 100g (3½oz) steamed brown rice (108)

■ **TOTAL MEAL:**

377

CALORIES

Grilled Ginger–Soy Chicken

Preparation time: 10 minutes / Marinating time: 2 hours
Cooking time: 20 minutes / Makes 8 servings

4tbsp reduced-sodium
   soy sauce
2tbsp fresh ginger,
   grated
2tbsp honey
2tbsp miso paste
1tbsp finely chopped
   garlic
2tsp toasted sesame
   oil
¼tsp chilli flakes
8 boneless, skinless
   chicken breast
   halves (1.4–1.8kg/
   3–4lb total)
½tsp flaky sea salt

MUFA: 120g (4¼oz)
   unsalted dry-
   roasted peanuts

1. In a large resealable plastic storage bag, combine the first seven ingredients. Add the chicken and turn to coat. Seal and chill for at least 2 hours.

2. Lightly coat a grill pan with vegetable oil spray. Heat the grill to medium for indirect heat. (If using a charcoal grill, position the coals on one half of grill. If using a gas grill, heat one side to high, the other to low.)

3. Remove the chicken from the marinade. Discard the marinade. Season the chicken with flaky sea salt.

4. Place the chicken on the hottest section of the grill. Cook for 10 minutes, turning once. Move to the cooler section of the grill and cook for 10 minutes or until a thermometer inserted into the thickest part of the chicken registers 74°C (165°F). Sprinkle with peanuts.

■ **Eat One Serving:**

317
CALORIES,
44g protein, 8g
carbohydrates, 12g
fat, 2g saturated
fat, 99mg
cholesterol, 424mg
sodium, 2g fibre

**MAKE IT A FLAT
BELLY DIET MEAL**
Serve with 150g
(5½oz) sliced red
peppers (40) with
2tbsp hummus for
dipping (50)

■ **TOTAL MEAL:**

407
CALORIES

Grilled Oregano Chicken

Preparation time: 10 minutes / Marinating time: 2 hours
Cooking time: 17 minutes / Makes 6 servings

6 small boneless,
    skinless chicken
    breast halves
    (about 1kg/2¼lb)
60g (2oz) coarsely
    chopped fresh
    oregano leaves
4 spring onions,
    trimmed and thinly
    sliced
120ml (4fl oz) balsamic
    vinegar

**MUFA: 90ml (6tbsp)
    extra virgin olive
    oil**

2tsp freshly ground
    black pepper
¾tsp salt

1. Place the chicken breast halves between 2 sheets of clingfilm. Using a mallet or heavy pan, pound to 2cm (¾in) thickness.

2. In a plastic resealable food storage bag, combine the oregano, spring onions, vinegar, oil, pepper and salt. Add the chicken, seal and turn to coat. Chill for 2 hours.

3. Lightly coat a grill pan with non-stick cooking spray. Preheat the grill to medium for indirect heat. (If using a gas grill, heat one side to high, the other to low.)

4. Remove the chicken from the marinade, reserving the marinade. Place the chicken on the hottest section of the grill. Cook for 10 minutes, turning once. Move the chicken to the cooler section of the grill and cook for 6 minutes more, turning once, until a thermometer inserted into the thickest part of the breast registers 74°C (165°F). Bring reserved marinade to boil for 5 minutes and pour over chicken.

■ **Eat One Serving:**

317

CALORIES,
40g protein, 5g
carbohydrates, 15g
fat, 2g saturated
fat, 99mg
cholesterol, 410mg
sodium, 0g fibre

**MAKE IT A FLAT
BELLY DIET MEAL**
Serve with 115g
(4oz) cherry
tomatoes (30) and
1 Laughing Cow®
Light wedge (35)

■ **TOTAL MEAL:**

382

CALORIES

Lime-Marinated Chicken with Salsa

Preparation time: 20 minutes / Marinating time: 1 hour
Cooking time: 13–15 minutes / Makes 4 servings

4 boneless, skinless
  chicken breast
  halves (about
  560g/1¼lb)
3tbsp lime juice (about
  3 limes)
2tbsp olive oil
1¼tsp ground cumin
¼tsp flaky sea salt
3 medium tomatoes,
  chopped

**MUFA: 1 medium
avocado, chopped**

90g (3oz) chopped
  mild onion
60g (2oz) chopped
  fresh coriander
1 small jalapeño
  chilli pepper,
  seeded and finely
  chopped

*Note: Wear plastic
gloves and keep hands
away from eyes when
handling fresh chilli
peppers.*

1. Put the chicken into a large resealable plastic bag.

2. In a small bowl, whisk the lime juice, oil, cumin and salt. Transfer 2 tablespoons of the marinade to a medium glass bowl and cover with clingfilm. Pour the remaining marinade into the chicken bag. Seal and turn to coat. Chill for at least 1 hour.

3. Meanwhile, add the tomatoes, avocado, onion, chopped coriander, and chilli pepper to the bowl with the lime marinade. Toss gently to mix. Cover the salsa and chill.

4. Coat the grill pan with non-stick cooking spray. Preheat the grill to medium–high. Cook the chicken, discarding the marinade, for 6 minutes on each side or until a thermometer inserted into thickest part of the chicken registers 74°C (165°F).

■ **Eat One Serving:**
307
CALORIES,
35g protein, 10g carbohydrates, 14.5g fat, 2g saturated fat, 82mg cholesterol, 249mg sodium, 4g fibre

MAKE IT A FLAT BELLY DIET MEAL
Serve on a bed of 115g (4oz) baby salad leaves (15) and 2 Ryvita® crispbreads (64)

■ **TOTAL MEAL:**
386
CALORIES

Chicken with Romesco Sauce

Preparation and cooking time: 30 minutes / Makes 4 servings

2 cloves garlic,
    crushed
1 slice firm whole grain
    bread, crust
    discarded and
    bread torn into
    pieces

**MUFA: 60g (2oz)
    slivered almonds**

230g (8oz) drained
    roasted red
    peppers (from a
    jar), coarsely
    chopped
1 tomato, seeded and
    coarsely chopped
1tbsp red-wine vinegar
1tsp smoked paprika
½tsp salt
2tbsp extra virgin oil
4 boneless, skinless
    chicken breast
    halves (145g/5oz
    each)

1. Toast the garlic and bread in a
large non-stick frying pan over
medium heat for 5 minutes or
until lightly browned, stirring
occasionally. Add the almonds
and continue cooking and
stirring for 3 minutes or until the
almonds are toasted. Transfer to
a food processor fitted with a
metal blade or a blender. Add
the peppers, tomato, vinegar,
paprika, salt and oil and purée.
Set aside.

2. Coat the same pan with
olive oil cooking spray and
return to medium heat. Add
the chicken and cook, turning
once, for 5 minutes or until
browned. Remove to a plate.
Add the reserved almond
mixture and bring to a simmer
over medium heat.

3. Return the chicken to the
pan. Cover and simmer for 10
minutes or until a thermometer
inserted in the thickest part
registers 74°C (165°F).

■ **Eat One Serving:**

340

CALORIES,
37g protein, 11g
carbohydrates, 16g
fat, 2g saturated
fat, 80mg
cholesterol, 430mg
sodium, 4g fibre

**MAKE IT A FLAT
BELLY DIET MEAL**
Serve with 170g
(6oz) steamed
asparagus (30)

■ **TOTAL MEAL:**

370

CALORIES

Almond-Encrusted Chicken Breast

Preparation time: 5 minutes / Cooking time: 10 minutes / Makes 1 serving

145g (5oz) boneless, skinless chicken breast
1tbsp cornflour
60ml (2fl oz) very low-fat egg substitute

MUFA: 2tbsp almonds, finely chopped

1. Sprinkle each side of the chicken breast with cornflour. Dip the breast into the egg substitute to coat and then sprinkle with almonds.

2. Coat a small non-stick frying pan with non-stick cooking spray and heat over medium heat. Cook the chicken for 5 minutes on each side or until a thermometer inserted in the thickest part registers 74°C (165°F).

■ **Eat One Serving:**

310

CALORIES,
43g protein, 10g carbohydrates, 9.8g fat, 1.5g saturated fat, 83mg cholesterol, 204mg sodium, 1g fibre

MAKE IT A FLAT BELLY DIET MEAL
Serve with 60g (2oz) very low-fat cottage cheese (40) and 115g (4oz) cherry tomatoes (30)

■ **TOTAL MEAL:**

380

CALORIES

Chicken Piccata

Preparation and cooking time: 15 minutes / Makes 4 servings

340g (12oz) boneless, skinless chicken fillets

2tbsp flour

MUFA: 4tbsp olive oil

2tbsp freshly squeezed lemon juice

2tbsp chopped fresh parsley

2tsp capers, minced

Freshly ground black pepper

1. Lay the chicken fillets on a work surface. With a rolling pin covered in clingfilm flatten to 5mm (¼in). Dredge the fillets lightly in the flour

2. Heat a large frying pan over medium–high heat. add the oil to the frying pan and heat until sizzling. Place the chicken in the pan. Cook for 2 minutes per side or until lightly browned and cooked through.

3. Add the lemon juice, parsley and capers. Bring the mixture to the boil. Reduce the heat and simmer for 2 minutes to allow the flavours to blend. Season to taste with the pepper. Serve the chicken with the pan juices.

Note: Pounding the chicken breasts to an even thickness is an important step because it allows the chicken to cook evenly so both ends are moist and delicious.

■ Eat One Serving:

235

CALORIES,

21g protein, 24g carbohydrates, 15g fat, 2g saturated fat, 49mg cholesterol, 108mg sodium, 0g fibre

MAKE IT A FLAT BELLY DIET MEAL

Serve with the Beetroot and Goat's Cheese Salad on p.164 (147)

■ TOTAL MEAL:

382

CALORIES

Chicken Pad Thai

Preparation and cooking time: 15 minutes / Makes 4 servings

115g (4oz) flat rice
    noodles
4tbsp ketchup
1tbsp fish sauce
1tsp sugar
1tbsp peanut
    (groundnut) oil,
    divided
1 egg, lightly beaten
340g (12oz) boneless,
    skinless cooked
    chicken breasts
    halves, cut into
    3cm (1½in) long
    strips
2 cloves garlic, finely
    chopped
3 spring onions, cut
    into 2.5cm (1in)
    pieces
45g (1½oz) bean
    sprouts

**MUFA: 60g (2oz)
unsalted peanuts,
finely chopped**

Lime wedges
    (optional)

1. Bring a pot of water to the boil and cook the noodles as per the packet instructions

2. Combine the ketchup, fish sauce and sugar in a small bowl. Heat 1 teaspoon of the peanut (groundnut) oil in a large non-stick frying pan over medium–high heat. Add the egg and cook, stirring occasionally, for about 2 minutes or until set. Transfer the egg to a bowl and reserve.

3. Return the pan to the cooker and heat the remaining 2 teaspoons oil, Add the chicken and cook, stirring often, for 4 to 5 minutes or until lightly browned and cooked through. Add the garlic and cook for 30 seconds longer. Stir in the noodles and cook for 1 minute longer or until hot. Add the ketchup mixture and cook, tossing, for 1 minute. Stir in the spring onions and remove from the heat.

4. Divide among 4 plates, garnishing each with 10g (¼oz) of the bean sprouts and sprinkling with the peanuts. Serve with the lime wedges, if desired.

■ **Eat One Serving:**

386

CALORIES,
29g protein, 36g carbohydrates, 15g fat, 2.5g saturated fat, 102mg cholesterol, 425mg sodium, 3g fibre

**A SINGLE SERVING
OF THIS RECIPE
COUNTS AS A
FLAT BELLY DIET
MEAL WITHOUT
ANY ADD-ONS!**

Slow Cooker Moroccan Chicken with Olives

Preparation and cooking time: 4–8 hours / Makes 6 servings

120ml (4fl oz) reduced-sodium chicken stock

45g (1½oz) plain flour

MUFA: 6tbsp olive oil

2tsp ground cumin

½tsp freshly ground black pepper

¼tsp salt

1 x 400g (14oz) tin tomatoes

1 carrot, sliced

1 large onion

30 small black olives, pitted

3 cloves garlic, finely chopped

900g (2lb) boneless, skinless chicken breast halves

60g (2oz) chopped fresh coriander (optional)

HARISSA

90g (3oz) dried hot red chilli peppers

2 cloves garlic, finely chopped

1tsp ground coriander

1tsp ground caraway seed

¼tsp salt

3tbsp olive oil

1. To prepare the chicken: coat the stoneware of a slow cooker pot with cooking spray. Combine the stock, flour, 3 tbsp oil, cumin, pepper and salt in the pot. Whisk until smooth. Add the tomatoes (with juice), carrot, onion, olives and garlic. Stir to mix. Tuck the chicken into the pot, covering with the other ingredients. Cover and cook on low for 5 to 6 hours or on high for 3 to 4 hours.

2. To prepare the harissa: remove the stems and seeds from the peppers and discard. Soak the peppers in warm water for about 1 hour or until softened. Drain and transfer to a food processor fitted with a metal blade or a blender. Add the garlic, coriander, caraway seed and salt. Process, scraping the sides of the bowl as needed, until a paste forms. Drizzle in the remaining oil through the tube to reach a smooth consistency.

3. Stir in the fresh coriander (if using) just before serving. Pass the harissa at the table.

■ **Eat One Serving:**

388

CALORIES,

38g protein, 16g carbohydrates, 19g fat, 3g saturated fat, 88mg cholesterol, 530mg sodium, 4g fibre

A SINGLE SERVING OF THIS RECIPE COUNTS AS A FLAT BELLY DIET MEAL WITHOUT ANY ADD-ONS!

Chicken with Honey Mustard and Pecan Topping

Preparation time: 10 minutes / Makes 2 servings

200g (7oz) boneless, skinless cooked chicken breasts or cooked chicken pieces

2tbsp reduced-fat sour cream

4tsp honey mustard

MUFA: 30g (1oz) pecans, toasted and chopped

1. Cut the chicken breasts into thin diagonal slices. Fan the slices out on 2 salad plates. Cut chicken into bite-size pieces.

2. In a small bowl, combine the sour cream and mustard. Stir to mix well. Dollop onto the chicken. Sprinkle with the pecans.

■ **Eat One Serving:**

307
CALORIES,

33g protein, 5g carbohydrates, 16g fat, 3g saturated fat, 90mg cholesterol, 120mg sodium, 1g fibre

MAKE IT A FLAT BELLY DIET MEAL
Serve on a bed of baby salad leaves (15) with 2 Ryvita® crispbreads (64)

■ **TOTAL MEAL:**

386
CALORIES

Zesty Chicken Fiesta

Preparation time: 5 minutes / Cooking time: 10 minutes / Makes 4 servings

284–340g (10–12oz) cooked chicken breast cut into chunks

420g (14½oz) tin low-salt black beans, rinsed and drained

400g (14oz) tin chopped tomatoes (with juice)

1tbsp chilli powder

MUFA: 1 medium avocado, chopped

60ml (2fl oz) sour cream, fat-free if available

1. In a non-stick frying pan, combine the chicken, beans, tomatoes and chilli powder. Bring the mixture to a simmer over medium–high heat. Reduce the heat to medium and cook, stirring occasionally, for about 5 minutes. Divide evenly among 4 salad plates and top each with ¼ of the avocado and 1 tablespoon of the sour cream.

■ **Eat One Serving:**

298

CALORIES,
30g protein, 26g carbohydrates, 8.5g fat, 1.5g saturated fat, 61mg cholesterol, 137mg sodium, 10g fibre

MAKE IT A FLAT BELLY DIET MEAL
Serve with 150g (5½oz) sliced red pepper (40) and 2tbsp hummus (50)

■ **TOTAL MEAL:**

388

CALORIES

Tuscan Chicken with Beans

Preparation time: 5 minutes / Makes 2 servings

170g (6oz) cooked, chopped chicken breast

200g (7oz) chopped tinned tomatoes flavoured with garlic and onion, drained

115g (4oz) tinned cannellini beans, rinsed and drained

2tsp balsamic vinegar

60g (2oz) salad leaves

MUFA: 30g (1oz) slivered almonds, toasted

1. In a bowl, toss together the chicken, tomatoes, beans and vinegar.

2. Divide the salad leaves between 2 salad plates and top each with 1/2 of the chicken mixture. Sprinkle with the almonds.

■ **Eat One Serving:**

294

CALORIES,

29g protein, 25g carbohydrates, 9.5g fat, 1g saturated fat, 54mg cholesterol, 112mg sodium, 9g fibre

MAKE IT A FLAT BELLY DIET MEAL

Serve with 50g (1³/₄oz) steamed wild rice (75)

■ **TOTAL MEAL:**

369

CALORIES

African Chicken Stew

Preparation and cooking time: 4–6 hours / Makes 4 servings

1tbsp peanut
   (groundnut) oil
340g (12oz) boneless,
   skinless chicken
   thighs, trimmed
   and cut into 24
   pieces
1 onion, chopped
3 cloves garlic, finely
   chopped
1 red chilli pepper,
   seeded and
   chopped
1 carrot, thickly sliced
1 sweet potato, peeled
   and cubed
420g (14½oz)
   reduced-sodium
   chicken stock

MUFA: 115g (4oz)
   crunchy natural
   unsalted peanut
   butter

2tbsp tomato paste
¼tsp salt
¼tsp freshly ground
   black pepper

1. Heat the oil in a large non-stick frying pan over medium-high heat. Add the chicken and cook, stirring occasionally, for 3 to 4 minutes or until lightly browned. Transfer to a 4 litre slow cooker. Return the frying pan to the heat and add the onion, garlic, chilli pepper and carrot. Cook for 1 minute, then transfer to the slow cooker. Stir in the sweet potato, stock, peanut butter and tomato paste.

2. Cook on high for 3 to 4 hours or low for 5 to 6 hours or until the chicken and vegetables are very tender. Season with salt and black pepper.

■ **Eat One Serving:**

439

CALORIES,
29g protein, 32g carbohydrates, 23g fat, 4g saturated fat, 71mg cholesterol, 615mg sodium, 7g fibre

A SINGLE SERVING OF THIS RECIPE COUNTS AS A FLAT BELLY DIET MEAL WITHOUT ANY ADD-ONS!

Steamed Salmon with Mangetout

Preparation time: 10 minutes / Cooking time: 12 minutes / Makes 4 servings

4 skinless salmon
fillets, about 3cm
(1½in) thick
(450-685g/1–1½lb)
1tsp grated fresh
ginger
1 clove garlic, finely
chopped
1tbsp freshly squeezed
lime juice (about 2
limes)
2tsp reduced-sodium
soy sauce
1tsp toasted sesame
oil
2 spring onions, thinly
sliced
450g (1lb) mangetout,
trimmed

**MUFA: 1 medium
avocado, chopped**

1. Rub the fillets with the ginger and garlic. Coat a steamer basket with non-stick cooking spray and arrange the fillets in the basket.

2. In a saucepan, bring 5cm (2in) of water to the boil. Place the steamer basket in the saucepan and cover. Cook for 8 minutes.

3. Meanwhile, in a small bowl, whisk together the lime juice, soy sauce, oil and spring onions. Set aside.

4. After the salmon has been cooking for 8 minutes, top with the mangetout and cover. Cook for about 4 minutes, until the salmon is opaque and the mangetout are tender but still crisp.

5. Make a bed of the mangetout on 4 plates, top with the salmon, sprinkle with the avocado, drizzle with the reserved sauce.

■ **Eat One Serving:**

330

CALORIES,

27g protein, 13g carbohydrates, 19g fat, 3.5g saturated fat, 67mg cholesterol, 176mg sodium, 6g fibre

**MAKE IT A FLAT
BELLY DIET MEAL**
Serve with 1 medium orange (70)

■ **TOTAL MEAL:**

400

CALORIES

Fish with Courgettes (Zucchini)

Preparation time: 8 minutes / Cooking time: 40 minutes / Makes 4 servings

1 large red onion,
    chopped, divided

**MUFA: 4tbsp extra
virgin olive oil,
divided**

1 strip lemon peel, cut
    into thin slivers
230g (8oz) courgettes
    (zucchini), cut into
    1cm (½in) chunks
230g (8oz) yellow
    courgettes
    (zucchini), cut into
    1cm (½in) chunks
1 clove garlic, finely
    chopped
4 striped bass fillets,
    about 2.5cm (1in)
    thick (450–685g/
    1–1½lb)
1tbsp red wine vinegar
1tbsp water
2tbsp finely chopped
    fresh mint

1. Preheat the oven to
200°C/400°F/gas 6. Set aside 2
tablespoons of the onion in a
small bowl. Place the remaining
onion in a 33 x 23cm (13 x 9in)
baking dish. Add 2 tablespoons
of the oil and the lemon peel.
Toss and then spread in an
even layer. Roast, stirring
occasionally, for about 15
minutes or until the onion is
tender. Remove the baking dish
from the oven. Stir in the
courgettes (zucchini) and
garlic. Roast for 10 minutes.
Remove from the oven.

2. Increase the oven
temperature to 230°C/450°F/
gas 8. Push the vegetables to
one side of the dish and add
the fish, arranging it evenly in
the pan. Top with the
vegetables. Roast until the fish
flakes easily with a fork (8 to
10 minutes for thin fillets; 12 to
15 minutes for thicker ones).

3. Meanwhile, add the vinegar,
water, mint and the remaining
2 tablespoons oil to the
reserved onion. Serve with the
fish.

■ **Eat One Serving:**

272

CALORIES,
22g protein, 8g
carbohydrates, 17g
fat, 2.5g saturated
fat, 91mg
cholesterol, 125mg
sodium, 2g fibre

**MAKE IT A FLAT
BELLY DIET MEAL**
Serve with 50g
(1¾oz) steamed
wild rice (75)

■ **TOTAL MEAL:**

347

CALORIES

Roast Fish with Artichokes

Preparation time: 10 minutes / Cooking time: 40 to 50 minutes
Makes 4 servings

2 large red onions, cut into 5mm (¼in) wedges

MUFA: 4tbsp extra virgin olive oil

285g (10oz) tinned artichoke hearts, drained

115g (4oz) small cherry tomatoes

2tbsp chopped parsley

1tsp freshly grated orange zest

1 clove garlic, finely chopped

4 skinless plaice fillets (450–685g/1–1½lb total)

1. Preheat the oven to 200°C/400°F/gas 6.

2. In a 32 x 23cm (13 x 9in) baking dish, combine the onions and oil. Toss and then spread in an even layer.

3. Roast for about 35 minutes or until the onions are very soft. Remove from the oven and stir in the artichokes and tomatoes.

4. In a small bowl, mix the parsley, orange zest and garlic. Set aside.

5. Increase the oven temperature to 230°C/450°F/gas 8. Push the vegetables to one side of the dish and add the fish, arranging it evenly in the pan. Spoon the vegetables over the fish and sprinkle with the parsley mixture.

6. Return the baking dish to the oven and roast until the fish flakes easily with a fork (about 5 minutes for thin fillets; 10 to 12 minutes for thicker fillets). Place the fillets on 4 plates.

■ **Eat One Serving:**

302

CALORIES,
24g protein, 15g carbohydrates, 16.5g fat, 2.5g saturated fat, 54mg cholesterol, 181mg sodium, 6g fibre

MAKE IT A FLAT BELLY DIET MEAL
Serve with 50g (1¾oz) steamed brown rice (50)

■ **TOTAL MEAL:**

352

CALORIES

Grilled Salmon Steak

Preparation time: 5 minutes / Marinating time: 30 minutes
Cooking time: 8 minutes / Makes 1 serving

MUFA: 1tbsp rapeseed (canola) oil

1tbsp freshly squeezed lemon juice (about ½ lemon)
Cayenne powder
½tsp chopped fresh dill
115g (4oz) salmon steak

1. In a resealable plastic bag, whisk the oil, lemon juice, cayenne pepper and dill. Add the salmon and massage the bag to coat evenly. Seal and chill for 30 minutes.

2. Preheat a grill to medium. Remove the salmon from the marinade. Pour the marinade into a microwaveable bowl. Cook the salmon under the grill for 4 minutes on each side or until opaque. Microwave the marinade on high power for about 1 minute or until boiling. Drizzle over the salmon.

■ **Eat One Serving:**

335

CALORIES,
23g protein, 1g carbohydrates, 26.5g fat, 3.5g saturated fat, 67mg cholesterol, 67mg sodium, 0g fibre

MAKE IT A FLAT BELLY DIET MEAL
Serve with baby salad leaves (15) tossed with 2tbsp Newman's Own® Light Balsamic Vinaigrette (45)

■ **TOTAL MEAL:**

395

CALORIES

Lemony Stuffed Sole

Preparation time: 10 minutes / Cooking time: 7 minutes / Makes 4 servings

450g (1lb) Dover sole fillets
¼tsp salt
⅛tsp freshly ground black pepper
230g (8oz) Courgette (Zucchini) Sauté (page 218)
1tsp extra virgin olive oil
60ml (2fl oz) dry white wine or 2tbsp freshly squeezed lemon juice mixed with 2tbsp vegetable stock
1tbsp butter
2tsp freshly squeezed lemon juice (about 1 lemon)
½tsp freshly grated lemon zest
1tsp finely chopped fresh parsley

MUFA: 60g (2oz) pumpkin seeds, toasted

1. Season both sides of the fish with salt and pepper. Place 1 fillet on a flat surface and spread 2 tablespoons of the courgette evenly over the top, leaving a 1cm (½in) margin on both ends. Roll the fillet into a cylinder and secure with wooden cocktail stick. Repeat with the remaining sole and courgette.

2. Heat the oil in a 30cm (12in) non-stick frying pan over medium heat and add the fish rolls, seam side up. Cook for 2 minutes. Add the wine or lemon juice–stock mixture. Reduce the heat to medium-low, cover and cook 5 minutes longer, or until the fish flakes easily with a fork.

3. Transfer the fish to a plate and tent loosely with aluminium foil. Add the butter, lemon juice and lemon zest to the frying pan. Remove from the heat, swirl until the butter melts and spoon over the fish. Remove the cocktail sticks from the fish and place each roll on a plate. Sprinkle with parsley and the pumpkin seeds.

■ **Eat One Serving:**

219

CALORIES,

24g protein, 8g carbohydrates, 9g fat, 3g saturated fat, 62mg cholesterol, 334mg sodium, 1g fibre

MAKE IT A FLAT BELLY DIET MEAL
Serve with 60g (2oz) skin-on cubed roast red potatoes (100) dressed with 2tbsp low-fat sour cream (40)

■ **TOTAL MEAL:**

359

CALORIES

Scallop Ceviche

Preparation time: 15 minutes / Chilling time: 1 hour / Makes 4 servings

230g (8oz) scallops

3tbsp finely chopped red onion

1 medium red chilli pepper, seeded and finely chopped (see Note)

Juice from 4 limes

30g (1oz) roughly chopped fresh coriander

1 small mango, stoned, peeled and diced

MUFA: 1 medium avocado, sliced

1. In a medium glass bowl, mix scallops, onion, chilli pepper and lime juice. Cover and chill for at least 1 hour. The scallops should be opaque to be edible in ceviche, but that does not mean they are 'cooked'. Handle any fish going into a ceviche with care.

2. Remove the scallop mixture from refrigerator. Drain the juice and discard. Mix in the coriander and mango. Divide the ceviche evenly among 4 plates. Fan out the avocado slices on the side.

Note: Wear plastic gloves and keep hands away from eyes when handling fresh chilli peppers.

■ **Eat One Serving:**

158

CALORIES,

11g protein, 18g carbohydrates, 6g fat, 1g saturated fat, 19mg cholesterol, 121mg sodium, 4g fibre

MAKE IT A FLAT BELLY DIET MEAL

Serve with 1 wholemeal pitta (140) and 1 apple (80)

■ **TOTAL MEAL:**

378

CALORIES

Chai Scallops with Pak Choi (Bok Choy)

Preparation time: 8 minutes / Cooking time: 12 minutes / Makes 4 servings

2 chai tea bags
2–4 heads baby pak choi (bok choy), quartered lengthways or halved if small (about 340g/12oz)
1tbsp finely chopped fresh ginger
450g (1lb) scallops, halved horizontally
¼tsp salt
2tsp rapeseed (canola) oil
80ml (3fl oz) light coconut milk

MUFA: 60g (2oz) cashews, chopped

1 lime, cut into 4 wedges

1. Bring 120ml (4fl oz) of water to the boil. Remove from the heat and steep the tea bags for 3 minutes. Remove and discard the tea bags. Reserve the brewed tea.

2. Sprinkle the pak choi (bok choy) with ginger. Steam over rapidly boiling water in a covered steamer for about 8 minutes or until bright green and easily pierced with the tip of a knife.

3. Pat the scallops dry and sprinkle with salt. Warm the oil in a large frying pan over medium–high heat. Add the scallops in a single layer. (Work in batches if necessary.) Cook for 2 minutes on each side or until opaque. Remove from the pan and set aside.

4. Add the tea and coconut milk to the frying pan. Cook for 1 to 2 minutes, swirling the pan and allowing the sauce to thicken. Divide the sauce evenly among 4 shallow bowls. Top with the pak choi (bok choy), scallops and cashews. Serve with the lime wedges.

■ **Eat One Serving:**
250
CALORIES,
23g protein, 12g carbohydrates, 12.5g fat, 3g saturated fat, 37mg cholesterol, 392mg sodium, 1g fibre

MAKE IT A FLAT BELLY DIET MEAL
Serve with 100g (3½oz) steamed wild rice (150)

■ **TOTAL MEAL:**
400
CALORIES

Sweet-and-Sour Prawns

Preparation time: 5 minutes / Cooking time: 6 minutes / Makes 2 servings

½tsp olive oil
230g (8oz) peppers,
     any colour, cut into
     strips
75g (2½oz) apricot
     jam
2tsp red wine vinegar
170g (6oz) cooked,
     peeled and
     deveined prawns

MUFA: 30g (1oz)
     unsalted dry-
     roasted peanuts,
     chopped

1. Heat the oil in a non-stick frying pan over medium–high heat. Add the peppers and cook, tossing, for about 3 minutes or until hot. Add the jam and vinegar. Cook for 1 minute or until bubbling. Add the prawns and cook for 2 minutes or until bubbling. Divide evenly between 2 plates and sprinkle with the peanuts.

■ **Eat One Serving:**

357

CALORIES,
23g protein, 44g carbohydrates, 11g fat, 1.5g saturated fat, 166mg cholesterol, 223mg sodium, 3g fibre

MAKE IT A FLAT BELLY DIET MEAL
Serve on a bed of 115g (4oz) baby salad leaves (15)

■ **TOTAL MEAL:**

372

CALORIES

Sizzled Prawns with Tomatoes

Preparation: time: 20 minutes / Cooking time: 12 minutes / Makes 4 servings

2tsp olive oil, divided
450g (1lb) large
    prawns, peeled
    and deveined
2tbsp finely chopped
    oil-packed
    sun-dried
    tomatoes
1 medium red onion,
    chopped
200g (7oz) sweetcorn
    kernels, cut from
    the cob (about 2
    medium cobs of
    corn)
3 medium tomatoes,
    chopped
4 cloves garlic, finely
    chopped
1/2tsp salt
1/4tsp freshly ground
    black pepper
30g (1oz) torn fresh
    basil leaves
30g (1oz) snipped
    fresh chives

**MUFA: 1 medium
    avocado, sliced**

1. Heat 1 teaspoon of the oil in large non-stick frying pan over medium–high heat. When hot, add the prawns and sizzle for 1 minute or until partially cooked. Transfer to small bowl.

2. Add the remaining 1 teaspoon oil to the frying pan along with the sun-dried tomatoes, onion and sweetcorn. Cook for 6 minutes or until the onion and sweetcorn are browned. Stir in the tomatoes and garlic. Cook for 3 minutes. Stir in the prawns and simmer for 1 to 2 minutes or until the prawns are opaque.

3. Season with the salt and pepper. Stir in the basil and chives. Spoon the prawn mixture into 4 shallow bowls. Garnish with the avocado.

■ **Eat One Serving:**

248

CALORIES,

22g protein, 21g carbohydrates, 10g fat, 1.5g saturated fat, 168mg cholesterol, 515mg sodium, 6g fibre

MAKE IT A FLAT BELLY DIET MEAL
Serve with 1 wholemeal pitta (140)

■ **TOTAL MEAL:**

388

CALORIES

Sesame Seared Scallops

Preparation time: 5 minutes / Cooking time: 10 minutes / Makes 4 servings

16 scallops (about
450g/1lb)
1/4tsp flaky sea salt
2tbsp very low-fat egg
substitute
40g (1 1/4oz) sesame
seeds
1tbsp peanut
(groundnut) oil
685g (1 1/2lb) baby pak
choi (bok choy)
(4–6 heads),
quartered
lengthways

**MUFA: 60g (2oz)
sunflower seeds**

1. Pat the scallops dry and
sprinkle both sides with salt.
Place the egg substitute in a
small bowl. Place the sesame
seeds on a small plate. Dip one
side of each scallop into the
egg substitute and then into
sesame seeds. Set aside.

2. Heat the oil in a large frying
pan over medium heat.
Arrange the scallops, sesame
side down, with space
between them, in the pan.
Cook for 3 to 4 minutes or until
the seeds are golden. Turn
each scallop carefully without
removing the sesame-seed
crust. Cook for 6 minutes
longer or until opaque.

3. Meanwhile, put the pak choi
(bok choy) into a steamer
basket set over a pot of boiling
water. Cover and steam for 6
minutes or until just tender.
Nestle the scallops among the
pak choi (bok choy) quarters
on each of 4 plates. Sprinkle
with the sunflower seeds.

■ **Eat One Serving:**

280

CALORIES,
20g protein, 11g
carbohydrates, 19g
fat, 2.5g saturated
fat, 20mg
cholesterol, 345mg
sodium, 5g fibre

**MAKE IT A FLAT
BELLY DIET MEAL**
Serve with
50g (1 3/4oz)
steamed
wild rice (75)

■ **TOTAL MEAL:**

355

CALORIES

Thai Sweet–Hot Prawns

Preparation time: 15 minutes / Marinating time: 30 minutes
Cooking time: 12 minutes / Makes 6 servings

3 cloves garlic, finely
    chopped
1 green chilli pepper,
    seeded and
    minced
    (see Note)
1½tbsp reduced-
    sodium fish sauce
    (*nam pla*) (see
    Note)
1½tbsp sugar
1tbsp freshly squeezed
    orange juice
1tbsp rice wine vinegar
½tsp chilli paste
685g (1½lb) large
    prawns, peeled,
    deveined and
    patted dry

**MUFA: 90g (3oz)
    unsalted dry-
    roasted peanuts,
    chopped**

1. In a small saucepan over medium heat, bring first seven ingredients to the boil. Reduce heat to medium and simmer for 3 minutes or until thickened slightly. Remove from the heat and let cool.

2. Place the prawns in a large bowl. Add 3 tablespoons of the cooled marinade, tossing well to coat. Cover and chill for 30 minutes.

3. Preheat a grill to medium–high. Coat the grill pan with non-stick cooking spray.

4. Thread the prawns on 6 metal skewers. Grill for 3 to 4 minutes, turning once, until opaque. Divide evenly among 4 plates and sprinkle with the peanuts.

Note: Wear plastic gloves and keep hands away from eyes when handling fresh chilli peppers.

Note: Reduced-sodium fish sauce – also called nam pla *– can be found in Asian supermarkets.*

■ **Eat One Serving:**

230

CALORIES,
25g protein, 9g carbohydrates, 11g fat, 1.5g saturated fat, 151mg cholesterol, 375mg sodium, 2g fibre

MAKE IT A FLAT BELLY DIET MEAL
Serve with 100g (3½oz) steamed wild rice (150)

■ **TOTAL MEAL:**

380

CALORIES

Seared Wild Salmon with Mango Salsa

Preparation time: 15 minutes / Marinating time: 1 hour
Cooking time: 15 minutes / Makes 6 servings

SALSA

1 ripe mango, stoned, peeled and diced
75g (2½oz) chopped red pepper, deseeded
75g (2½oz) chopped red onion
3tbsp freshly squeezed lime juice
2tbsp chopped fresh mint
1tbsp finely chopped red chilli pepper (see Note)
¼tsp salt

SALMON

60ml (2fl oz) freshly squeezed lemon juice (about 2 lemons)
½tsp paprika
¼tsp salt
2 wild salmon fillets (about 900g/2lb, 2.5cm (1in) thick)
1tbsp olive oil

MUFA: 240g (8½oz) avocado, mashed

1. To prepare the salsa: In a small bowl, toss together the mango, pepper, onion, lime juice, mint, chilli pepper and salt. Cover and chill for at least 1 hour to blend flavours.

2. To prepare the salmon: in a large shallow baking dish, combine the lemon juice, paprika and salt. Place the salmon in the dish and turn to coat both sides. Marinate, covered, for up to 1 hour in refrigerator.

3. Remove the fillets from the marinade. Discard the marinade. Heat the oil in a large non-stick frying pan over medium–high heat. Sear the fillets for 15 minutes, turning once or until opaque. On each of 6 plates, place ⅓ fillet of salmon topped with ⅓ of the salsa and avocado.

Note: Wear plastic gloves and keep hands away from eyes when handling fresh chilli peppers.

■ **Eat One Serving:**

364

CALORIES,
32g protein, 15g carbohydrates, 20.5g fat, 3g saturated fat, 83mg cholesterol, 267mg sodium, 5g fibre

A SINGLE SERVING OF THIS RECIPE COUNTS AS A FLAT BELLY DIET MEAL WITHOUT ANY ADD-ONS!

Dijon Pork Loin Chops with Cabbage

Preparation time: 18 minutes / Cooking time: 36 minutes / Makes 4 servings

4 pork loin chops
    (about 450g/1lb),
    trimmed
4tsp Dijon mustard
1tsp plus 1tbsp
    rapeseed (canola)
    oil
1tbsp grated fresh
    ginger
½tsp ground
    cinnamon
¼tsp ground cloves
½ head red cabbage
    (about 450g/1lb),
    cored and
    shredded
2 Granny Smith
    apples, peeled and
    grated
1tbsp maple syrup
¼tsp salt
2tsp cider vinegar

**MUFA: 60g (2oz)
    pumpkin seeds,
    toasted**

1. Brush both sides of the chops with mustard and set aside. In a large heavy frying pan with a lid, warm 1 teaspoon of the oil over medium-low heat. Add the ginger, cinnamon and cloves. Cook, stirring, for 10 to 15 seconds. Add the cabbage, apples, maple syrup and salt. Stir, reduce the heat to low, cover and cook for about 30 minutes.

2. Meanwhile, in a heavy frying pan, heat remaining 1 tablespoon oil over medium-high heat. Arrange chops in a single layer. Cook, turning halfway through, for about 9 minutes or until a thermometer inserted in the centre of a chop registers 68°C (155°F).

3. Add the vinegar to the cabbage mixture. Increase the heat to medium. Cook for about 5 minutes or until most of the liquid evaporates. Place each chop on a plate with a mound of the cabbage mixture. Sprinkle with the pumpkin seeds.

■ **Eat One Serving:**

316
CALORIES,
28g protein, 25g carbohydrates, 12.5g fat, 2.5g saturated fat, 70mg cholesterol, 317mg sodium, 4g fibre

MAKE IT A FLAT BELLY DIET MEAL
Serve with 50g (1¾oz) steamed brown rice (55)

■ **TOTAL MEAL:**

371
CALORIES

Mexican Pork Tenderloin

Preparation time: 10 minutes / Marinating time: 12 hours
Cooking time: 30 minutes / Makes 4 servings

½ medium onion, chopped
3 cloves garlic, finely chopped
2 fresh chilli peppers, finely chopped
3tbsp cider vinegar
2tbsp orange juice
1tbsp sugar
2tsp rapeseed (canola) oil
1tsp chopped fresh oregano
685g (1½lb) pork tenderloin
½tsp ground cumin
½tsp salt
¼tsp freshly ground black pepper

MUFA: 1 medium avocado, sliced

1. Coat a small frying pan with cooking spray and cook the onion and garlic over medium-high heat for 5-7 minutes. Purée in a blender with the chilli peppers, vinegar, orange juice, sugar, oil and oregano. Place the pork in a shallow dish and cover with the paste. Cover and refrigerate overnight.

2. Preheat a grill to medium-high for indirect heat. (If using a charcoal grill, push the coals to one side. If using a gas grill, heat one side to high, the other to medium.)

3. In a small bowl, combine the cumin, salt and black pepper. Remove the pork from the marinade and blot dry with a paper towel. Rub with the cumin mixture. Grill the pork for 10 minutes. Move to the cooler section of the grill. Cover and grill for 10 minutes more or until a thermometer inserted in the centre reaches 68°C (155°F). Let it stand for 10 minutes before slicing. Divide the slices evenly among 4 plates and top with the avocado.

■ **Eat One Serving:**

329

CALORIES,
37g protein, 11g carbohydrates, 15g fat, 3g saturated fat, 111mg cholesterol, 416mg sodium, 3g fibre

MAKE IT A FLAT BELLY DIET MEAL
Serve with 115g (4oz) cherry tomatoes (30)

■ **TOTAL MEAL:**

359

CALORIES

Stir-Fried Rice with Asian Vegetables and Beef

Preparation time 15 minutes / Cooking time 12 minutes / Makes 4 servings

285g (10oz) brown rice

1 sirloin steak (230g/8oz, 2cm/¾in thick), thinly sliced

2tbsp reduced-sodium soy sauce, divided

2tsp rapeseed (canola) oil

400g (14oz) fresh or frozen Asian vegetable mix or stir-fry vegetables

1tbsp finely chopped fresh ginger

2tsp finely chopped garlic

5 diagonally sliced spring onions

MUFA: 60g (2oz) dry-roasted unsalted peanuts, coarsely chopped

1. Cook the rice according to the packet directions. Set aside.

2. Meanwhile, in a bowl, combine the steak with 1 tablespoon of the soy sauce. Toss to mix. Heat a wok or large frying pan over high heat. Add the oil. Place the steak in a single layer and cook without stirring, for 1 minute, to brown. Cook for 1 more minute, stirring once or twice, until all the pink in the meat is gone. With a slotted spoon or tongs, transfer the meat to a clean dish and set aside. Add the frozen vegetables to the pan. Cook over medium heat, stirring constantly, for about 5 minutes or until the vegetables are tender.

3. Add the ginger and garlic to the pan and stir-fry for 30 seconds. Add the steak, spring onions, peanuts, rice and the remaining 1 tablespoon soy sauce. Cook, stirring, for about 2 minutes or until heated through.

■ **Eat One Serving:**

330

CALORIES,

21g protein, 30g carbohydrates, 15g fat, 2.5g saturated fat, 27mg cholesterol, 356mg sodium, 5g fibre

MAKE IT A FLAT BELLY DIET MEAL

Serve with 1 medium orange (70)

■ **TOTAL MEAL:**

400

CALORIES

Vietnamese Beef Salad

Preparation time: 15 minutes / Marinating time: 30 minutes
Cooking time: 8–10 minutes / Makes 4 servings

60ml (2fl oz) reduced-sodium soy sauce
60ml (2fl oz) freshly squeezed lime juice (about 2 limes)
60ml (2fl oz) water
2tbsp sugar
1tbsp garlic, finely chopped
2tsp chilli paste
230g (8oz) braising steak
400g (14oz) mixed salad leaves
60g (2oz) fresh basil
60g (2oz) fresh coriander
2 large red onions, thinly sliced
2 large seedless cucumbers, with peel, cut in long, thin strips
4 medium carrots, cut in long, thin strips

MUFA: 60g (2oz) unsalted dry-roasted peanuts, chopped

1. In a medium bowl, whisk together the first six ingredients. Pour 3 tablespoons into a resealable plastic storage bag. Cover and refrigerate the remaining dressing. Add the steak to the bag, seal and turn to coat. Chill for 30 minutes.

2. Heat a grill to medium–high heat. Grill the steak for 8 to 10 minutes, turning once or until a thermometer inserted sideways in the centre registers 63°C (145°F) for medium–rare. Let it rest for 5 minutes and slice thinly at an angle across the grain.

3. In a large bowl, combine the salad leaves, basil and coriander. Divide the salad mixture evenly among 4 plates. Sprinkle on the onions, cucumbers and carrots. Top each salad with the sliced steak, drizzle with the dressing and sprinkle with peanuts.

■ **Eat One Serving:**

323

CALORIES,
22g protein, 30g carbohydrates, 14.5g fat, 3g saturated fat, 21mg cholesterol, 654mg sodium, 8g fibre

MAKE IT A FLAT BELLY DIET MEAL
Serve with 115g (4oz) red grapes (60)

■ **TOTAL MEAL:**

383

CALORIES

Basic Balsamic Braising Steak

Preparation time: 5 minutes / Marinating time: 1 hour
Cooking time: 16 minutes / Makes 4 servings

685g (1½lb) braising
  steak
150ml (5fl oz) balsamic
  vinegar
1tbsp freshly ground
  black pepper
2 cloves garlic

MUFA: 4tbsp olive oil

1. Prick the meat with a fork to help the marinade penetrate. Mix the remaining ingredients in a large resealable bag. Drop the steak into the bag, seal and refrigerate for 1 hour or up to 24 hours.

2. Preheat a grill to medium for direct heat. Remove the meat from the bag, reserving the marinade. Grill the meat for 6 to 8 minutes per side or until a thermometer inserted into the thickest part registers 63°C (145°F) for medium–rare. In a small saucepan, boil the reserved marinade for 5 minutes.

3. Slice the meat diagonally across the grain in thin slices and drizzle with the marinade. Divide evenly among 4 plates.

■ **Eat One Serving:**

393

CALORIES,
37g protein, 7g carbohydrates, 23g fat, 5.5g saturated fat, 56mg cholesterol, 108mg sodium, 0g fibre

A SINGLE SERVING OF THIS RECIPE COUNTS AS A FLAT BELLY DIET MEAL WITHOUT ANY ADD-ONS!

Broccoli and Tofu Stir-Fry with Toasted Almonds

Preparation time: 30 minutes / Cooking time: 12 minutes / Makes 4 servings

230g (8oz) broccoli
florets

450g (1lb) extra-firm
tofu, diced

3tsp toasted sesame
oil, divided

1 bunch spring onions
(about 8), trimmed
and thinly sliced

3 cloves garlic, finely
chopped

1 small jalapeño chilli
pepper, seeded
and finely
chopped (see
Note)

3½tsp low-sodium soy
sauce

**MUFA: 60g (2oz)
sliced almonds,
lightly toasted**

400g (14oz) cooked
brown rice

1. Lightly steam the broccoli for about 5 minutes or until tender but still crisp. Set aside.

2. Heat 2 teaspoons of the oil in a wok or large non-stick frying pan over high heat. When hot, add the tofu and cook, stirring constantly, for 5 minutes or until browned. Transfer to a shallow bowl.

3. Add the remaining 1 teaspoon oil to the wok. Heat for 30 seconds. Add the spring onions, garlic, chilli pepper and broccoli. Stir-fry over medium–high heat for 2 minutes. Stir in the soy sauce, almonds and tofu, tossing gently to combine. Divide the stir-fry and brown rice evenly among 4 plates.

Note: Wear plastic gloves and keep hands away from eyes when handling fresh chilli peppers.

■ **Eat One Serving:**

360

CALORIES,

21g protein, 33g carbohydrates, 18g fat, 2.5g saturated fat, 0mg cholesterol, 184mg sodium, 7g fibre

MAKE IT A FLAT BELLY DIET MEAL

Serve with 150g (5½oz) sliced red pepper (40)

■ **TOTAL MEAL:**

400

CALORIES

Chickpea Salad

Preparation time: 5 minutes / Cooking time: 18 minutes / Makes 4 servings

1tbsp olive oil
½ medium onion, chopped
2 cloves garlic, finely chopped
1tsp curry powder
½ medium yellow pepper, seeded and chopped
2 x 400g (14oz) tins chopped tomatoes
1 x 450g (1lb) tin chickpeas rinsed and drained
60g (2oz) fresh or tinned pineapple, chopped
115g (4oz) thinly sliced fresh spinach

MUFA: 1 medium avocado, mashed

1. Heat the oil in a large non-stick frying pan over medium heat. Add the onion, garlic and curry powder. Cook, stirring occasionally, for about 3 minutes, or until the onion starts to soften.

2. Add the pepper, tomatoes, chickpeas and pineapple. Reduce the heat to medium–low and simmer for 10 to 15 minutes, or until heated through. Stir in the spinach during the last 5 minutes of cooking. Divide evenly among 4 plates and top with ¼ of the avocado.

■ **Eat One Serving:**

278

CALORIES,
7g protein, 35g carbohydrates, 13g fat, 2g saturated fat, 0mg cholesterol, 319mg sodium, 10g fibre

MAKE IT A FLAT BELLY DIET MEAL
Serve with 100g (3½oz) cooked brown whole grain rice (110)

■ **TOTAL MEAL:**

388

CALORIES

Courgette (Zucchini) Fusilli

Preparation time: 5 minutes / Cooking time: 10 minutes / Makes 2 servings

40g (1¼oz) wholemeal fusilli pasta or any other short shape of pasta

170g (6oz) very low-fat cottage cheese

1tbsp Italian herb seasoning

60g (2oz) shredded courgettes (zucchini)

200g (7oz) tinned chopped tomatoes, drained

30g (1oz) reduced-fat shredded mozzarella cheese

MUFA: 20 medium black olives, sliced

1. Prepare the pasta according to the packet directions. Drain and set aside.

2. In a microwaveable dish, combine the cottage cheese and Italian seasoning. Stir in the pasta and courgettes (zucchini). Top with tomatoes and sprinkle with mozzarella. Microwave on high for 3 minutes to warm through. Divide the pasta evenly between 2 plates and sprinkle with the olives.

■ **Eat One Serving:**

223

CALORIES,

18g protein, 20g carbohydrates, 8g fat, 2.5g saturated fat, 12mg cholesterol, 864mg sodium, 4g fibre

MAKE IT A FLAT BELLY DIET MEAL

Serve with 4 ounces sliced turkey, rolled up (100), and 150g (5½oz) sliced red pepper (40)

■ **TOTAL MEAL:**

363

CALORIES

Vegetable Stew

Preparation time: 10 minutes / Cooking time: 20 minutes / Makes 4 servings

MUFA: 4tbsp extra virgin olive oil

1 large onion, chopped
3 cloves garlic, finely chopped
450g (1lb) tinned whole tomatoes
½tsp dried thyme
⅛tsp salt
450g (1lb) green beans, trimmed and cut into 5cm (2in) pieces
1 medium courgette (zucchini), halved and sliced
30g (1oz) chopped fresh basil

1. Heat the oil in a large non-stick frying pan over medium heat. Add the onion and garlic and cook, stirring occasionally, for 4 minutes or until tender.

2. Add the tomatoes (with juice), thyme and salt, stirring to break up the tomatoes. Bring to the boil over high heat. Add the green beans. Reduce the heat to low, cover and simmer, stirring occasionally, for 10 minutes or until the beans are tender.

3. Add the courgette (zucchini) and cook, stirring occasionally, for 5 minutes, or until tender. Remove from the heat and stir in the basil.

■ Eat One Serving:

194
CALORIES,
4g protein, 18g carbohydrates, 14g fat, 2g saturated fat, 0mg cholesterol, 242mg sodium, 7g fibre

MAKE IT A FLAT BELLY DIET MEAL
Serve with 90g (3oz) grilled chicken breast (90) and 50g (1¾oz) steamed wild rice (75)

■ TOTAL MEAL:

359
CALORIES

Stir-Fried Broccoli and Mushrooms with Tofu

Preparation time: 10 minutes / Cooking time: 8 minutes / Makes 4 servings

80ml (3fl oz) vegetable stock

1tbsp apricot all-fruit spread

1tbsp reduced-sodium soy sauce

1tbsp dry sherry

2tsp cornflour

1tbsp rapeseed (canola) oil

1 large head broccoli, cut into florets

4 cloves garlic, finely chopped

1tbsp grated fresh ginger

115g (4oz) fresh mushrooms, sliced

115g (4oz) cherry tomatoes

230g (8oz) firm tofu, cubed

MUFA: 60g (2oz) cashews, toasted and chopped

1. In a cup, whisk together first five ingredients. Set aside.

2. Heat the oil in a large non-stick frying pan over medium–high heat. Add the broccoli, garlic and ginger and cook for 1 minute. Add the mushrooms and cook, stirring frequently, for 3 minutes or until the broccoli is tender but still crisp.

3. Add the tomatoes and tofu, and cook, stirring frequently, for 2 minutes or until the tomatoes begin to collapse.

4. Stir the cornflour mixture and add to the frying pan. Cook, stirring, for 2 minutes or until the mixture thickens. Divide evenly among 4 plates and sprinkle with the cashews.

■ **Eat One Serving:**

283

CALORIES,

16g protein, 25g carbohydrates, 16g fat, 2.5g saturated fat, 0mg cholesterol, 246mg sodium, 6g dietary fibre

MAKE IT A FLAT BELLY DIET MEAL

Serve with 1 medium orange (70)

■ **TOTAL MEAL:**

353

CALORIES

Penne with Mushrooms and Artichokes

Preparation and cooking time: 20 minutes / Makes 4 servings

170g (6oz) whole wheat penne pasta

1tbsp extra virgin olive oil

230g (8oz) sliced white mushrooms

1 onion, chopped

3 cloves garlic, finely chopped

540g (18oz) cherry tomatoes

400g (14oz) tinned artichoke hearts, drained and chopped

MUFA: 4tbsp pesto, shop-bought

4tsp grated Romano cheese

1. Bring a large pot of lightly salted water to the boil. Add the penne and cook as per the packet directions. Drain.

2. Meanwhile, heat the oil in a large non-stick frying pan over medium–high heat. Add the mushrooms and onion and cook, stirring occasionally, for 7 to 8 minutes or until the mushrooms have released their liquid and start to brown slightly. Add the garlic and cook for 1 minute longer. Stir in the tomatoes and artichokes and cook for another 1 to 3 minutes or until the tomatoes just begin to soften.

3. Add the pasta and toss to combine. Remove from the heat and stir in the pesto.

4. Divide among 4 bowls and top each with 1 teaspoon of the cheese.

■ **Eat One Serving:**

370

CALORIES,

16g protein,
49g carbohydrates,
13g fat, 2g saturated fat,
5mg cholesterol,
790mg sodium,
6g fibre

MAKE IT A FLAT BELLY DIET MEAL

Have ½ medium pear as a dessert (52)

■ **TOTAL MEAL:**

422

CALORIES

Soya Beans with Sesame and Spring Onions

Preparation time: 6 minutes / Cooking time: 14 minutes / Makes 4 servings

340g (12oz) frozen, shelled green soya beans (edamame)
1tbsp soy sauce
120ml (4fl oz) water

MUFA: 60g (2oz) slivered almonds

Dash hot pepper sauce (optional)
2 spring onions, finely chopped
1½tsp toasted sesame oil
⅛tsp freshly ground black pepper

1. In a medium saucepan over high heat, bring the soya beans, soy sauce and water to the boil, stirring occasionally. Reduce the heat to low and simmer for 12 minutes or until tender. If any liquid remains, cook, stirring occasionally, over medium–high heat until the liquid has evaporated.

2. Remove from the heat. Stir in the almonds, hot pepper sauce (if using), spring onions, oil and pepper. Divide evenly among 4 plates.

■ **Eat One Serving:**

212

CALORIES,

13g protein, 12g carbohydrates, 13.5g fat, 1.5g saturated fat, 0mg cholesterol, 340mg sodium, 6g fibre

MAKE IT A FLAT BELLY DIET MEAL
Serve with 100g (3½oz) steamed wild rice (150)

■ **TOTAL MEAL:**

362

CALORIES

Balsamic Roasted Carrots

Preparation time: 5 minutes / Cooking time: 25 minutes / Makes 2 servings

8 medium carrots,
quartered
lengthways

**MUFA: 2tbsp extra
virgin olive oil,
divided**

1tbsp balsamic vinegar
½tsp salt
¼tsp freshly ground
black pepper

1. Preheat oven to 230°C/450°F/gas 8.

2. In a roasting pan, combine the carrots, 2 tablespoons oil, vinegar, salt and pepper. Toss to coat. Roast for 20 to 25 minutes, tossing occasionally, until lightly caramelized and tender but still firm.

■ **Eat One Serving:**

177

CALORIES,
1g protein, 12g carbohydrates, 14.5g fat, 2g saturated fat, 0mg cholesterol, 356mg sodium, 3g fibre

MAKE IT A FLAT BELLY DIET MEAL
Serve with organic mixed baby salad leaves (16), 115g (4oz) halved cherry tomatoes (30), and 1 wholemeal pitta (140)

■ **TOTAL MEAL:**

363

CALORIES

Brown Rice Pilaf with Mushrooms

Preparation and cooking time: 1 hour 20 minutes / Makes 4 servings

240ml (8fl oz)
     reduced-sodium
     fat-free chicken or
     vegetable stock
120ml (4fl oz) water

**MUFA: 60g (2oz)
     pecans**

1½tbsp olive oil
1 large onion, halved
     and finely sliced
2 cloves garlic, finely
     chopped
285g (10oz) baby
     portobello
     mushrooms,
     quartered
½tsp allspice
½tsp dried thyme
⅛tsp salt
⅛tsp freshly ground
     black pepper
145g (5oz) short- or
     long-grain brown
     rice

1. Preheat the oven to 180°C/350°F/gas 4. Combine the stock and water in a small saucepan and bring to the boil over high heat. Set aside.

2. Toast the pecans in a large non-stick frying pan over medium heat, stirring often, for about 3 to 4 minutes or until lightly browned and fragrant. Tip onto a plate.

3. Heat the oil in a large flameproof saucepan or casserole with a lid over medium heat. Add the onion and garlic. Cover and cook, stirring often, for about 6 minutes or until tender.

4. Stir in the mushrooms, thyme, allspice, pepper and salt (the pan will seem dry). Cover and cook, stirring often, for about 6 minutes or until the mushrooms have released their liquid and the liquid has evaporated. Stir in the rice and pecans.

5. Add the reserved stock mixture and bring to the boil. Cover and transfer to the oven. Bake for about 50 to 60 minutes or until the rice is tender and the liquid has been absorbed. Let stand for 5 minutes before fluffing with a fork and serving.

■ **Eat One Serving:**

311

CALORIES,
7g protein, 37g carbohydrates, 16g fat, 2g saturated fat, 0mg cholesterol, 265mg sodium, 4g fibre

TO SERVE AS PART OF ANOTHER FLAT BELLY DIET MEAL
Omit the pecans and serve with 75g (2½oz) Roast Fish with Artichokes, p.194 (110)

■ **TOTAL MEAL:**

421

CALORIES

Courgette (Zucchini) Sauté

Preparation time: 10 minutes / Cooking time: 45 minutes / Makes 8 servings

2tbsp extra virgin olive oil
6 cloves garlic, sliced
1tsp chilli flakes
1.4kg (3lb) assorted courgettes (zucchini), green and yellow, thinly sliced into discs
½tsp salt

MUFA: 120g (4¼oz) sunflower seeds

1. In a large non-stick frying pan set over medium heat, combine the oil, garlic and chilli flakes. Cook, stirring occasionally, for 2 to 3 minutes or until the garlic begins to turn golden. Add the courgettes (zucchini) and salt. Toss to coat. Cover, reduce the heat to medium–low and cook for 30 minutes, stirring occasionally, until the courgettes begin to break apart.

2. Uncover the pan and increase the heat to medium. Cook for 10 to 12 minutes longer or until the liquid is almost gone. Divide evenly among 8 plates and sprinkle with the sunflower seeds.

■ **Eat One Serving:**

156

CALORIES,
5g protein, 10g carbohydrates, 12g fat, 1.4g saturated fat, 0mg cholesterol, 156mg sodium, 4g fibre

MAKE IT A FLAT BELLY DIET MEAL
Serve with 4 ounces roasted turkey, rolled up (100), 150g (5½oz) sliced red pepper (40), and 4tbsp hummus (100)

■ **TOTAL MEAL:**

396

CALORIES

Wild Rice with Almond and Cranberry Dressing

Preparation time: 15 minutes / Standing time: 10 Minutes
Cooking time: 1 hour, 15 minutes / Makes 8 servings

230g (8oz) wild rice
2 strips (1 x 5cm/½ x 2in) orange peel
1 stick celery, 8cm (3in) of leafy top only
2tsp salt
1.5l (2 ½ pints) water
2 whole cloves
½ small onion, plus 2 medium chopped onions
1tbsp olive oil
2 cloves garlic, finely chopped
230g (8oz) seedless green grapes
115g (4oz unsweetened dried cranberries
240ml (8fl oz) low-sodium chicken stock
30g (1oz) chopped flat-leaf parsley

MUFA: 120g (4¼oz) sliced almonds, toasted

1. In a deep, wide 5-litre casserole over high heat, bring rice, orange peel, celery, salt and water to the boil. Stick the cloves into the onion half and add to the casserole. Cover and cook over medium–low heat for 35 to 45 minutes or until the rice is tender. Remove from the heat and let it stand, covered, for 10 minutes. Remove and discard the orange peel, onion with cloves and celery. Set aside.

2. Heat the oil in a large frying pan over medium heat and add the chopped onions. Reduce the heat to low, cover and cook for 5 minutes. Increase the heat to medium. Uncover and cook, stirring occasionally, for about 10 minutes. Add the garlic and cook for 1 minute. Add the onion mixture, grapes, cranberries, stock and parsley to the rice and stir to blend. Cover and cook over low heat for 15 minutes. Sprinkle with the almonds.

■ **Eat One Serving:**

322

CALORIES,

9g protein, 56g carbohydrates, 8.5g fat, 1g saturated fat, 0mg cholesterol, 655mg sodium, 6g fibre

MAKE IT A FLAT BELLY DIET MEAL
Serve with 1 apple (80)

■ **TOTAL MEAL:**

402

CALORIES

Guilt-Free Chips

Preparation time: 5 minutes / Cooking time: 25 minutes / Makes 4 servings

1 large sweet potato and 1 large Maris Piper potato (685g/1½lb total), peeled and sliced into thin strips

MUFA: 4tbsp rapeseed (canola) oil

½tsp chilli powder
½tsp garlic powder
½tsp ground cumin
½tsp sea salt

1. Preheat the oven to 230°C/450°F/gas 8.

2. In a bowl, toss together the potatoes, oil, chilli powder, garlic powder and cumin. Arrange the potatoes in a single layer on a baking sheet. Bake for 25 minutes. Halfway through, turn the chips over and continue baking.

3. Remove the chips from the oven and place them on several layers of paper towels. Sprinkle with the salt.

■ **Eat One Serving:**

243

CALORIES,

3g protein, 28g carbohydrates, 14g fat, 1g saturated fat, 0mg cholesterol, 338mg sodium, 3g fibre

MAKE IT A FLAT BELLY DIET MEAL

Serve with 115g (4oz) mixed baby salad leaves (15) and 115g (4oz) halved cherry tomatoes (30) tossed with 2tbsp Newman's Own® Light Balsamic Vinaigrette (45) and 115g (4oz) sweetcorn (70)

■ **TOTAL MEAL:**

403

CALORIES

Stir-Fried Asparagus with Ginger, Sesame and Soya

Preparation time: 5 minutes / Cooking time: 12 minutes / Makes 4 servings

685g (1½lb) asparagus, trimmed and cut into 5cm (2in) pieces

MUFA: 4tbsp rapeseed (canola) oil

½ large red pepper, seeded and cut into strips

1tbsp chopped fresh ginger

1tbsp reduced-sodium soy sauce

⅛tsp chilli flakes

2tsp toasted sesame oil

1tsp sesame seeds

1. Bring 5mm (¼in) water to the boil in a large non-stick frying pan over high heat. Add the asparagus and return to the boil. Reduce the heat to low, cover and simmer for 5 minutes or until tender but still crisp. Drain in a colander and cool briefly under cold running water. Wipe the frying pan dry with a paper towel.

2. Heat the rapeseed (canola) oil in the same frying pan over high heat. Add the pepper and cook, stirring constantly, for 3 minutes, or until tender but still crisp. Add the asparagus, ginger, soy sauce and chilli flakes and cook for 2 minutes, or until heated through. Remove from the heat and stir in the sesame oil and the sesame seeds.

■ **Eat One Serving:**

190

CALORIES,

4g protein, 9g carbohydrates, 17g fat, 1.5g saturated fat, 0mg cholesterol, 145mg sodium, 4g fibre

MAKE IT A FLAT BELLY DIET MEAL

Serve with 115g (4oz) roasted turkey, rolled up (100), 115g (4oz) cherry tomatoes (30), and 1 medium orange (70)

■ **TOTAL MEAL:**

390

CALORIES

Tuscan White Bean Spread

Preparation time: 10 minutes / Makes 12 servings

420g (14½oz) tinned cannellini or haricot beans, rinsed and drained
1 large clove garlic
1tbsp freshly squeezed lemon juice (about 1 lemon)
2tsp white wine vinegar
2 sprigs fresh flat-leaf Italian parsley
2 basil leaves
1tsp Dijon mustard
¼tsp dried oregano
Chilli flakes

MUFA: 180ml (6fl oz) olive oil

Salt
Freshly ground black pepper

1. In a food processor bowl fitted with a metal blade or in a blender, combine the beans, garlic, lemon juice, vinegar, parsley, basil, mustard, oregano and chilli flakes to taste. Purée until smooth.

2. With the processor or blender running, slowly pour in the oil until it is all absorbed. Season to taste with salt and black pepper.

■ **Eat One Serving:**

140

CALORIES,
1g protein, 4g carbohydrates, 13.5g fat, 2g saturated fat, 0mg cholesterol, 87mg sodium, 1g fibre

MAKE IT A FLAT BELLY DIET MEAL
Serve with 1 wholemeal pitta (140) and 115g (4oz) cherry tomatoes (30)

■ **TOTAL MEAL:**

310

CALORIES

Plum and Nectarine Trifle

Preparation time: 35 minutes / Standing time: 30 minutes / Chilling time: 1 hour / Makes 6 servings

3 plums, stoned and
    thinly sliced
2 nectarines, stoned
    and thinly sliced
60g (2oz) honey
1tbsp raspberry or
    white balsamic
    vinegar
230g (8oz) low-fat
    vanilla yogurt
230g (8oz) low-fat
    ricotta cheese, if
    available
1 fat-free trifle sponge
    (285g/10oz), cut
    into 1cm (1/2in)
    slices

**MUFA: 90g (3oz)
slivered almonds,
toasted**

1. In a medium bowl, toss the plums and nectarines with the honey and vinegar. Let it stand for 30 minutes at room temperature, stirring once or twice.

2. In a small bowl, whisk together the yogurt and ricotta until smooth.

3. Line the bottom of a 2-litre clear glass serving bowl with half of the cake slices. Sprinkle on some of the juice from the fruit. Spread half of the fruit over the cake. Sprinkle on half of the almonds. Spoon on half of the yogurt mixture. Use the remaining cake slices to make a second layer. Top with the remaining fruit. Spoon on the remaining yogurt mixture to cover the fruit. Decorate the top with the remaining almonds.

4. Cover with clingfilm and chill for 1 hour or up to 24 hours before serving.

■ **Eat One Serving:**

371

CALORIES,
13g protein, 62g carbohydrates, 10g fat, 2.5g saturated fat, 15mg cholesterol, 289mg sodium, 4g fibre

Chocolate Strawberries

Preparation time: 3 minutes / Cooking time: 8 minutes
Cooling time: 30 minutes / Makes 4 servings

**MUFA: 180g (6¼oz)
dark chocolate
chips**

1tbsp skimmed milk
20 ripe medium
strawberries with
stalks

1. Line a baking tray with parchment paper.

2. Place the chocolate and milk in the top of a double boiler or bain marie set over boiling water. Reduce the heat to medium and allow the chocolate to melt, about 3 minutes. Stir until the mixture is smooth. Remove from the heat.

3. Holding by the stem, dip each berry into chocolate, coating three-quarters of the way up. Place on the parchment, leaving 2.5cm (1in) of space around each berry.

4. Chill for 30 minutes to set the chocolate.

■ **Eat One Serving:**

222

CALORIES,

2g protein, 31g carbohydrates, 13g fat, 7.5g saturated fat, 0mg cholesterol, 7mg sodium, 4g fibre

MAKE IT A FLAT BELLY DIET MEAL

Serve with 230g (8oz) very low-fat cottage cheese (160) sprinkled with cinnamon

■ **TOTAL MEAL:**

382

CALORIES

Irresistible Brownies

Preparation time: 35 minutes / Makes 8 servings

75g (2½oz)
    unbleached plain
    flour
50g (1¾oz)
    unsweetened cocoa
    powder, sifted if
    lumpy
¼tsp baking powder
⅛tsp salt
130 (4½oz) packed
    dark brown sugar
4tbsp canola oil
1 large egg + 1 large
    egg white
1tsp vanilla extract
30g (1oz) dark
    chocolate chips

**MUFA: 120g (4¼oz)
walnuts**

1. Preheat oven to 180°C/
350°F/gas 4. Coat a 20 x 20cm
(8 x 8in) baking pan with
cooking spray.

2. Combine the flour, cocoa,
baking powder and salt in a
large bowl.

3. Combine the brown sugar,
oil, egg and egg white, and
vanilla extract in a small bowl.
Whisk until smooth. Pour into
the flour mixture and stir until
blended. Stir in the chocolate
chips and walnuts (the batter
will be stiff).

4. Spread the batter in a thin
layer in the prepared pan.
Bake for 20 to 22 minutes or
until firm at the edges and a
wooden cocktail stick inserted
off centre comes out with a
few moist crumbs. Place pan
on a rack and let cool
completely. Cut into 8 bars.

■ **Eat One Serving:**

305

CALORIES,

5g protein, 31g
carbohydrates, 22g
fat, 2g saturated
fat, 26mg
cholesterol, 75mg
sodium, 2g fibre

**MAKE IT A FLAT
BELLY DIET MEAL**

Serve with 1 scoop
reduced-fat vanilla
ice cream (100)

■ **TOTAL MEAL:**

405

CALORIES

Oat Cookies with Cranberries and Chocolate Chips

Preparation time: 10 minutes / Baking time: 10 minutes / Makes 24 cookies

230g (8oz) rolled oats

75g (2½oz) wholemeal plain flour

¾tsp bicarbonate of soda

½tsp ground cinnamon

¼tsp salt

90g (3oz) brown sugar

80ml (3fl oz) rapeseed (canola) oil

3 large egg whites

2tsp vanilla extract

90g (3oz) cranberries, coarsely chopped

MUFA: 360g (13oz) chopped walnuts

60g (2oz) dark chocolate chips

1. Preheat the oven to 180°C/350°F/gas 4. In a large bowl, combine the oats, flour, baking soda, cinnamon and salt.

2. In a medium bowl, whisk together the brown sugar, oil, egg whites and vanilla extract until smooth. Fold in the cranberries, walnuts and chocolate chips. Gradually fold in the flour mixture and stir until well blended.

3. Drop the batter by tablespoons onto 2 large baking trays coated with non-stick cooking spray. Bake for 10 minutes or until the cookies are golden brown.

4. Transfer the cookies to a wire rack to cool completely.

■ **Eat One Serving:**

172

(1 cookie):
CALORIES,
4g protein, 15g carbohydrates, 11.8g fat, 1.5 g saturated fat, 0mg cholesterol, 73mg sodium, 2g fibre

MAKE IT A FLAT BELLY DIET MEAL
Serve with 115g (4oz) cottage cheese (80) and 1 medium apple (80)

■ **TOTAL MEAL:**

332

CALORIES

Chocolate Pudding with Bananas and Digestive Biscuits

Preparation time: 5 minutes / Cooking time: 5 minutes / Chilling time: 2 hours / Makes 6 servings

3 whole digestive
    biscuits, crushed
1 ripe banana, sliced
90g (3oz) sugar
4tbsp unsweetened
    cocoa powder
3tbsp cornflour
Salt
700ml (1¼ pints)
    skimmed milk
½tsp vanilla extract

MUFA: 270g (9½oz) dark chocolate chips

1. Evenly divide the digestive biscuit crumbs among 6 ramekins. Press the crumbs to cover the bottoms of the ramekins. Top with the banana slices, reserving some for garnish.

2. In a large saucepan, mix the sugar, cocoa, cornflour and salt. Stir in the milk. Whisk over medium heat for about 4 minutes or until the pudding comes to the boil and thickens.

3. Cook for 1 minute longer. Remove from the heat and stir in the vanilla extract. Pour into the prepared ramekins. Chill for at least 2 hours, or until set.

4. Sprinkle each custard with ¼ of the chocolate chips and the reserved banana slices.

■ **Eat One Serving:**

391

CALORIES,

7g protein, 65g carbohydrates, 15g fat, 8.5g saturated fat, 10mg cholesterol, 147mg sodium, 4g fibre

A SINGLE SERVING OF THIS RECIPE COUNTS AS A FLAT BELLY DIET MEAL WITHOUT ANY ADD-ONS!

Red Fruit Crumble

Preparation time: 1 hour / Makes 6 servings

FRUIT

450g (1lb)
strawberries, hulled
and thickly sliced

3 ripe plums, cut into
2.5cm (1in) pieces

145g (5oz) fresh or
frozen raspberries

60g (2oz) all-fruit
raspberry or
strawberry
preserve, stirred
smooth

TOPPING

30g (1oz) oatmeal

45g (1½oz) wholemeal
plain flour

4tbsp firmly packed
dark brown sugar

½tsp ground
cinnamon

⅛tsp salt

3tbsp trans-fat-free
margarine, cut into
small pieces

**MUFA: 90g
(3oz)chopped
walnuts**

1. Preheat the oven to
180°C/350°F/gas 4.

2. To prepare the fruit:
combine the strawberries,
plums, raspberries and fruit
preserve in a 20 x 20cm (8 x
8in) glass baking dish and mix
gently with a spatula.

3. To prepare the topping: mix
the oats, flour, brown sugar,
cinnamon and salt in a
medium bowl, crumbling the
mixture with your hands to
break up the lumps of sugar.
Add the margarine and
crumble until well
incorporated. Stir in the
walnuts. Sprinkle over the
fruit.

4. Bake, uncovered, for 35 to
40 minutes or until the fruit is
tender and bubbly and the
topping is lightly browned.
Place the baking dish on a rack
and let it cool for at least 30
minutes before serving.

■ **Eat One Serving:**

332

CALORIES,

6g protein, 46g
carbohydrates, 14g
fat, 1.5g saturated
fat, 0mg
cholesterol, 95mg
sodium, 6g fibre

**MAKE IT A FLAT
BELLY DIET MEAL**

Serve with 115g
(4oz) reduced-fat
vanilla ice cream
(100)

■ **TOTAL MEAL:**

432

CALORIES

The-Best-for-Last Chocolate Mousse

Preparation time: 10 minutes / Makes 4 servings

340g (12oz) soft silken tofu, drained
2tsp vanilla extract
¼tsp almond extract

MUFA: 180g (6¼oz) dark chocolate chips, melted

115g (4oz) fat-free Greek-style yogurt

1. Place the tofu, vanilla and almond extracts in a food processor and blend until smooth. Add the chocolate and blend for 1 minute. Scrape the sides with a rubber spatula and blend for 1 minute longer or until incorporated. Pour into a large bowl.

2. Fold in the yogurt just until blended. Refrigerate until ready to serve.

Note. For chocolate semifreddo, place the mixture in a 23cm (9in) loaf tin lined with foil. Cover and freeze for 3 to 4 hours or until just set. Serve immediately.

■ **Eat One Serving:**

350

CALORIES,
11g protein, 40g carbohydrates, 18g fat, 10g saturated fat, 0mg cholesterol, 15mg sodium, 4g fibre

MAKE IT A FLAT BELLY DIET MEAL
Serve with fresh raspberries (30).

■ **TOTAL MEAL:**

380

CALORIES

READ A FLAT BELLY
SUCCESS
STORY

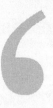

Nichole Michl

AGE: 46

POUNDS LOST:

12

IN 32 DAYS

ALL-OVER INCHES LOST:

11

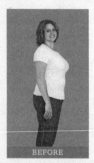
BEFORE

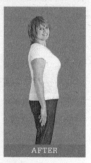
AFTER

I LOST 12 POUNDS IN 1 MONTH PLUS 3½ INCHES AROUND THE waist! I was thrilled!' exclaims Nichole Michl.

And well she should be. The 46-year-old graphic designer had tried to lose weight off and on over the years and had even been successful at times. But she could never seem to get rid of her belly fat. 'That was always the last to go,' she laments. And it was the most annoying to her. So she thought, *'If this* Flat Belly Diet *does what its name says it's going to do – if it's going to help me get rid of my belly fat – I'm going to be one very happy woman.'*

Nichole already knew this about herself: when she makes a commitment to something – especially a public commitment – she's more likely to follow it through. So, she challenged herself. 'I made the decision to go on the diet – all 32 days' worth – and then I told everyone I knew, so there was no backing out.'

She's also the kind of person who, if she commits to something, does it 100 per cent. She followed the rules to the letter, she says. 'Every single thing they said to do, I did. I bought the right foods. I measured everything. I even followed the diet when I was out, because I know that when you go to a friend's house for dinner, it's so easy to let your guard down – you know, "I'll try it just this once". Then, before you know it, you've blown it.'

Determined not to let that happen, if Nichole ate at a restaurant, or even if she went away for a weekend, she took along her food in a coolbox. 'I recently went to a picnic where 50 people sat around eating burgers and other stuff from the barbecue, and there I was with my little container of food and my bottle of water,' she says. 'And I looked at what they were eating and what *I* was eating, and I was fine with it. Particularly because so much of what I was eating was organic, and I know that's healthy for me.'

Nichole calls the support she had during those 32 days a key to her success. Cheered on the whole way by her family and colleagues, she revelled in her weight loss. 'You couldn't help but see the changes in my body,' she says, 'which made me want to keep going. Plus, it was great knowing they were all on my side.'

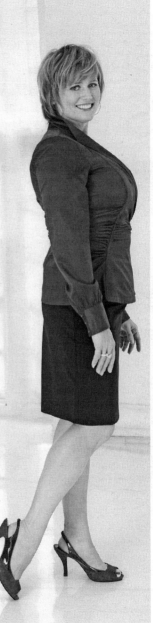

Being on the diet slowed her down in what she says is a good way. 'I had a tendency to eat really quickly – just to get it over with. Like at work. I know you're not supposed to do this, but I always ate at my desk. When I started the diet, though, I learned to pace myself. I thought about what I was eating and truly appreciated every morsel. Even the portions of nuts. Instead of popping a handful of nuts in my mouth at once, I'd bite off a piece of one, chew it and really savour it. I try now to do that with everything.' She plans to continue with the diet. With this kind of weight loss plus a flatter belly – it's a life plan.

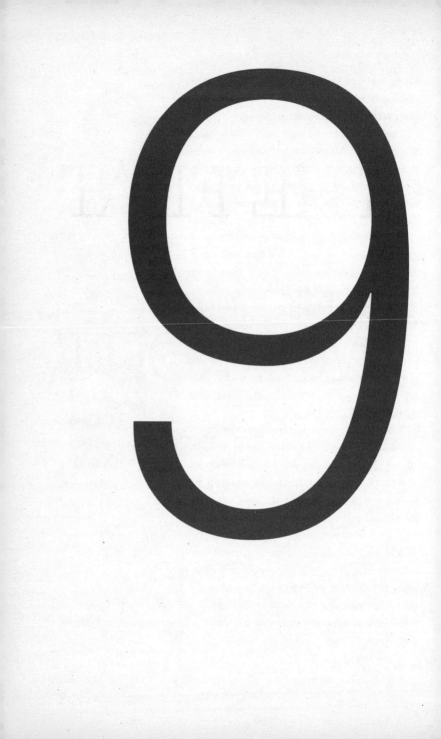

THE FLAT BELLY WORKOUT

THREE YEARS AGO, after nearly 2 months of doctor-prescribed bed rest followed by a Caesarean section and the birth of my two daughters, Sophia and Olivia, I was desperate to move again. Pre-babies, I had exercised all the time, sometimes devoting 10 to 15 hours a week to working out. I'd run five mornings a week, then walk to work and often do a lunchtime strength-training class at the gym. I religiously attended Thursday night yoga classes for years. (As a friend once said, 'When you don't have kids, your day can be as long as you want it to be.')

Then the girls came along, and my whole concept of 'me' time changed – for ever. Once I was back at work, I had far too much to pack into my 9-hour day to squeeze in a lunchtime workout. Mornings were out: I was up at 5.30 a.m. and racing to catch an early train.

Yoga classes after work? I dashed out every day at 5.15 to get home in time to spend an hour with my girls before they went to bed. Bottom line: I still needed to exercise, but between an hour-a-day commute, children and a full-time job, it was simply impossible to keep up my pre-pregnancy schedule.

I know from experience how difficult it can be to fit exercise into a busy life. That's why it was important to me that the *Flat Belly Diet* should include a workout plan that could be tailored to fit any schedule. Even though this diet plan is designed to provide results if you don't exercise, every expert I know firmly believes in the power of aerobic exercise and strength training to boost your mood and energy levels, as well as help you prevent disease and maintain bone and muscle mass as you age. Of course, it will also deliver faster results if you're following the *Flat Belly Diet*, as was demonstrated with our test panellists. Those who added daily exercise lost, on average, 70 per cent more body weight and 25 per cent more inches than the non-exercisers. While *every single one* of our testers lost fat and inches around their middles – even those who just followed the eating plan – the exercisers lost more and lost it faster.

A Routine Grounded in Science

WHEN I ASKED fitness director Michele Stanten to devise a companion workout plan for the *Flat Belly Diet*, I knew she'd start by looking for a plan that was backed by the most current research and delivered results. Just like the eating plan, this exercise plan had to be what I call 'life-proof'. I didn't want any drama attached to it – no running out to buy this or that piece of wacky equipment, no clearing out your cellar and turning it into a Pilates studio, no working out madly for months at a time, dreaming of the day you can just lie down in a deckchair and finally relax. It had to be a programme that most women would find enjoyable and do-able within the context of their already busy and demanding schedules. Oh, and I had one more directive for Michele: no crunches.

I don't know anyone who loves crunches. All that straining on your neck and lower back, all that huffing and puffing . . . it just doesn't add up. And if the truth were told, they're not that effective. In all the research we've seen come out of the exercise labs, the crunch is *never* the move that is found to target ab muscles the best. Over the years, I've met top trainers with the most incredibly defined mid-sections who tell me they moved on from crunches a decade ago. Today, the truly evolved fitness trainers develop belly-centric workouts that don't focus on just one set of ab muscles but target your whole core – front, sides and back.

The Flat Belly Workout Basics

THE FLAT BELLY Workout is built around three main components:

- Cardio exercise to burn calories and shed fat
- Strength training with weights to build muscle and boost metabolism
- Core-focused exercises to tone and tighten your mid-section

The first part of the plan, **cardio exercise**, burns calories, which is the only way to shrink the layer of fat covering your tummy muscles. Unless you're shedding that fat, you can spend hours doing ab exercises without seeing a change. I recommend walking for aerobic exercise because it's easy and accessible and offers loads of benefits, but you can do anything you like: cycling,

The Exercise Bonus

In a study published in the *Journal of Clinical Endocrinology and Metabolism*,[1] obese post-menopausal women with type 2 diabetes were split into three groups. One group was given a low-calorie diet high in MUFAs that included a nutrition consultation and weekly support meetings. Another group followed a supervised aerobic exercise programme consisting of 50-minute walks, three times a week. The third group received both programmes. After 14 weeks, the diet-only and exercise-plus-diet groups lost similar amounts of weight, about 10lb, but the combined group lost nearly twice as much visceral belly fat.

The Dynamic Duo

If you're going to exercise, I urge you to do both strength training and aerobic exercise. If you're a walker, try the strength exercises in this chapter. If you're all-weights-all-the-time, then add our suggested aerobic routine to your life. The right mix of cardio and strength exercise is important for fast, lasting results. In one study, women in their forties did either straight aerobic exercise (60 minutes, 6 days a week) or a mix of workouts (60 minutes of aerobic exercise, 3 days a week and 60 minutes of strength training, 3 days a week[2]). After 24 weeks, the combined training group lost 40 per cent more weight, three times more subcutaneous fat and – most important – 12 per cent more dangerous visceral fat. Even better, they also increased lean body mass such as muscle that fuels your metabolism.

swimming, jogging, or using machines like treadmills, stair climbers and elliptical trainers.

I'm recommending two types of cardio walks: **Fat Blast** and **Calorie Torch Walks**. Fat Blast walks are steadily paced walks guaranteed to burn off belly fat. The length of these walks will increase each week, and as you become more fit, you should be able to walk at a faster pace (and burn fat faster!) without feeling any extra effort. Calorie Torch walks are set up to be executed in intervals, meaning periodic bursts of fast-paced walking interspersed with a moderate pace. Studies show that interval training keeps metabolism revved up long after the workout is done. The upshot? You burn more calories throughout the day.

If you can't fit in all six cardio workouts every week, don't beat yourself up: just do what you can. I want you to customize the workouts so they fit your lifestyle. If you're like me, you'll be much more likely to stick with something that you a) *enjoy* and b) *can actually do*. These days, I'm more about walking and hiking (I can bring my daughters along) rather than the spinning classes I attended religiously in my thirties. It's all about what works for you, right now, at this point in your life.

In addition to the daily walk, you'll also be following a strength-training regime – either **The Metabolism Boost** or **The Belly Routine**.

The Metabolism Boost workout includes four combined moves that target multiple body parts – like your arms and legs – simultaneously. At the same time, they burn more calories overall and in less time (love that). Each of these moves also has a balance challenge, so while you're working your arms, legs, buttocks, chest and back, your core will be constantly engaged. Let me repeat that: *even while you're doing the metabolism-boosting moves, you will be working the muscles of your belly.*

The Belly Routine is nothing less than the best and most effective crunch-free exercise routine ever devised. All of the suggested moves have been lab-tested and shown to be up to 80 per cent more effective than traditional crunches.

These workouts are designed to tone and tighten not only your abs but every inch of your body. So wave goodbye to those jiggly trouble spots on your legs, buttocks and arms, along with your belly. The beauty of these strength routines is that each has only four or five moves – the most effective ones based on research – so you can get firm fast. You should aim to do three of each weekly. But as I said earlier, if that's not possible, even one or two of each of these routines a week will help to speed up your results. If you do all six workouts one week, make sure to take one rest day each week. It doesn't matter what day you choose; feel free to work it around your schedule.

EXERCISE TIP

If you plan to exercise and have to skip one workout, don't skip **The Metabolism Boost**. In the short term, these are the exercises that will translate into higher calorie burning all day long. Maintaining muscle is essential for preserving lean body mass.

The Importance of Speed and Intensity

IF YOU WANT to lose your belly fat, your 'walk' must be aerobic enough to get your heart pumping. That's where speed and intensity factor in. The programme we've set out for you incorporates both *steady-paced* and *interval* walks. The steady-paced **Fat Blast** walks are just that. You'll walk at a constant, brisk speed for a certain amount of time, gradually increasing the duration as shown in the plan. And, as you become fitter and your muscles get stronger, you'll naturally walk faster and burn more calories, without it feeling any harder. For instance, a 2-mile walk at 2mph burns 170 calories (based on a 10stone 10lb person). But when you ratchet it up to 3mph in that same hour, you'll burn 224 calories – a third more calories, and not an extra minute of exercise time. A win–win situation, don't you agree?

When you do the interval walks – aka **Calorie Torch** walks – you'll be alternating brisk-paced bouts with faster, higher-intensity bursts. In both cases, you can start with the level that is the most comfortable for you and work your way up as you gain more endurance.

Intensity refers to the level at which you perform your exercise. What is high intensity for someone who has not exercised before may be low intensity for someone who works out on a regular basis. No matter what your fitness level, you can achieve a high-intensity workout simply by pushing yourself just a little out of your comfort zone.

Working at high intensity can burn from 25 to 75 per cent more calories than exercising at low intensity. Running, biking, even step aerobics all work the same way. The faster you go or the more effort it takes (say, for example, you're heading up a steep hill), the greater the benefits. You'll be evaluating your level of intensity on a 1-to-10 scale: 1 being how you feel when you're sitting on the couch and 10

EXERCISE TIP
Stay Hydrated. Drink at least 2 glasses of water about 2 hours before your workout, and then about ½ glass every hour during exercise.

being how you'd feel sprinting as fast as you can. It's impossible – and unhealthy – to maintain an extremely high intensity for an entire workout. It's most effective to push yourself into this zone in spurts. Here's how the levels break down:

	HOW IT FEELS	INTENSITY LEVEL	SPEED (MPH) *
WARM-UP, COOL-DOWN	Easy enough that you can sing	3–4	3.0–3.5
BRISK	You can talk freely, but no more singing	5–6	3.5–4.0
FAST	You can talk in brief phrases, but you'd rather not	7–8	4.0+

* Note that these walking speeds are merely guidelines. The fitter you get, the faster you'll walk at each of these levels.

Use these pace and exertion levels (based on a 1-to-10 scale) to ensure that you're working out at the right intensity level for your Fat Blast and Calorie Torch walks.

■ FAT BLAST – Steady-paced walks burn off belly fat. Walk at a brisk speed (5–6 intensity level).

■ CALORIE TORCH – Interval walks raise your calorie burn during and after your workout to shed even more belly fat. Alternate brisk walking (5–6 intensity level) with short bursts of fast walking (7–8 intensity level).

(continued on page 244)

Your One-Month Walking Plan

DAY 1

Fat Blast Walk

TOTAL WORKOUT TIME	HOW IT BREAKS DOWN	INTENSITY LEVEL
30 minutes	3 min warm-up	3–4
	25 min brisk	5–6
	2 min cool-down	3–4

DAY 2

Calorie Torch Walk

TOTAL WORKOUT TIME	HOW IT BREAKS DOWN	INTENSITY LEVEL
25 minutes	3 min warm-up	3–4
	4 min brisk	5–6
	1 min fast	7–8
	(do brisk/fast intervals 4 times)	
	2 min cool-down	3–4

DAY 3

Fat Blast Walk

TOTAL WORKOUT TIME	HOW IT BREAKS DOWN	INTENSITY LEVEL
30 minutes	3 min warm-up	3–4
	25 min brisk	5–6
	2 min cool-down	3–4

DAY 4

Calorie Torch Walk

TOTAL WORKOUT TIME	HOW IT BREAKS DOWN	INTENSITY LEVEL
25 minutes	3 min warm-up	3–4
	4 min brisk	5–6
	1 min fast	7–8
	(do brisk/fast intervals 4 times)	
	2 min cool-down	3–4

DAY 5

Fat Blast Walk

TOTAL WORKOUT TIME	HOW IT BREAKS DOWN	INTENSITY LEVEL
30 minutes	3 min warm-up	3–4
	25 min brisk	5–6
	2 min cool-down	3–4

DAY 6

Calorie Torch Walk

TOTAL WORKOUT TIME	HOW IT BREAKS DOWN	INTENSITY LEVEL
25 minutes	3 min warm-up	3–4
	4 min brisk	5–6
	1 min fast	7–8
	(do brisk/fast intervals 4 times)	
	2 min cool-down	3–4

DAY 7

REST

Fat Blast Walk

DAY 1	TOTAL WORKOUT TIME	HOW IT BREAKS DOWN	INTENSITY LEVEL
	45 minutes	3 min warm-up	3-4
		40 min brisk	5-6
		2 min cool-down	3-4

Calorie Torch Walk

DAY 2	TOTAL WORKOUT TIME	HOW IT BREAKS DOWN	INTENSITY LEVEL
	35 minutes	3 min warm-up	3-4
		4 min brisk	5-6
		1 min fast	7-8
		(do brisk/fast intervals 6 times)	
		2 min cool-down	3-4

Fat Blast Walk

DAY 3	TOTAL WORKOUT TIME	HOW IT BREAKS DOWN	INTENSITY LEVEL
	45 minutes	3 min warm-up	3-4
		40 min brisk	5-6
		2 min cool-down	3-4

Calorie Torch Walk

DAY 4	TOTAL WORKOUT TIME	HOW IT BREAKS DOWN	INTENSITY LEVEL
	35 minutes	3 min warm-up	3-4
		4 min brisk	5-6
		1 min fast	7-8
		(do brisk/fast intervals 6 times)	
		2 min cool-down	3-4

Fat Blast Walk

DAY 5	TOTAL WORKOUT TIME	HOW IT BREAKS DOWN	INTENSITY LEVEL
	45 minutes	3 min warm-up	3-4
		40 min brisk	5-6
		2 min cool-down	3-4

Calorie Torch Walk

DAY 6	TOTAL WORKOUT TIME	HOW IT BREAKS DOWN	INTENSITY LEVEL
	35 minutes	3 min warm-up	3-4
		4 min brisk	5-6
		1 min fast	7-8
		(do brisk/fast intervals 6 times)	
		2 min cool-down	3-4

DAY 7	
	REST

Fat Blast Walk

	TOTAL WORKOUT TIME	HOW IT BREAKS DOWN	INTENSITY LEVEL
DAY 1	60 minutes	3 min warm-up 55 min brisk 2 min cool-down	3–4 5–6 3–4

Calorie Torch Walk

	TOTAL WORKOUT TIME	HOW IT BREAKS DOWN	INTENSITY LEVEL
DAY 2	45 minutes	3 min warm-up 4 min brisk 1 min fast (do brisk/fast intervals 8 times) 2 min cool-down	3–4 5–6 7–8 3–4

Fat Blast Walk

	TOTAL WORKOUT TIME	HOW IT BREAKS DOWN	INTENSITY LEVEL
DAY 3	60 minutes	3 min warm-up 55 min brisk 2 min cool-down	3–4 5–6 3–4

Calorie Torch Walk

	TOTAL WORKOUT TIME	HOW IT BREAKS DOWN	INTENSITY LEVEL
DAY 4	45 minutes	3 min warm-up 4 min brisk 1 min fast (do brisk/fast intervals 8 times) 2 min cool-down	3–4 5–6 7–8 3–4

Fat Blast Walk

	TOTAL WORKOUT TIME	HOW IT BREAKS DOWN	INTENSITY LEVEL
DAY 5	60 minutes	3 min warm-up 55 min brisk 2 min cool-down	3–4 5–6 3–4

Calorie Torch Walk

	TOTAL WORKOUT TIME	HOW IT BREAKS DOWN	INTENSITY LEVEL
DAY 6	45 minutes	3 min warm-up 4 min brisk 1 min fast (do brisk/fast intervals 8 times) 2 min cool-down	3–4 5–6 7–8 3–4

DAY 7	REST

Fat Blast Walk

DAY 1	TOTAL WORKOUT TIME	HOW IT BREAKS DOWN	INTENSITY LEVEL
	60 minutes	3 min warm-up 55 min brisk 2 min cool-down	3–4 5–6 3–4

Calorie Torch Walk

DAY 2	TOTAL WORKOUT TIME	HOW IT BREAKS DOWN	INTENSITY LEVEL
	45 minutes	3 min warm-up 4 min brisk 1 min fast (do brisk/fast intervals 8 times) 2 min cool-down	3–4 5–6 7–8 3–4

Fat Blast Walk

DAY 3	TOTAL WORKOUT TIME	HOW IT BREAKS DOWN	INTENSITY LEVEL
	60 minutes	3 min warm-up 55 min brisk 2 min cool-down	3–4 5–6 3–4

Calorie Torch Walk

DAY 4	TOTAL WORKOUT TIME	HOW IT BREAKS DOWN	INTENSITY LEVEL
	45 minutes	3 min warm-up 4 min brisk 1 min fast (do brisk/fast intervals 8 times) 2 min cool-down	3–4 5–6 7–8 3–4

Fat Blast Walk

DAY 5	TOTAL WORKOUT TIME	HOW IT BREAKS DOWN	INTENSITY LEVEL
	60 minutes	3 min warm-up 55 min brisk 2 min cool-down	3–4 5–6 3–4

Calorie Torch Walk

DAY 6	TOTAL WORKOUT TIME	HOW IT BREAKS DOWN	INTENSITY LEVEL
	45 minutes	3 min warm-up 4 min brisk 1 min fast (do brisk/fast intervals 8 times) 2 min cool-down	3–4 5–6 7–8 3–4

DAY 7

REST

Get Your Walking Form Up to Speed

THE SECRET TO turning your everyday stroll into a fat-blasting stride is proper walking form and technique. The most common mistake people make when they try to pick up the pace is that they take longer strides. This can actually slow you down because your outstretched leg acts like a brake, and it can cause injuries due to increased stress on your joints. Instead, take shorter, quicker steps, rolling from heel to toes and pushing off with your toes. Next, bend your arms at about 90-degree angles and swing them forwards (no higher than chest height) and back so your hand is almost skimming your hip. Letting your arms flail across your body will slow down your forward momentum. Practise these techniques and you'll be cruising past other walkers in no time.

Gear Up for Your Walks

YOUR SHOES

■ **Find a knowledgeable salesperson.** Unlike mass-market retailers, speciality stores often employ trained shoe fitters who will ask you about your walking habits and watch you walk. This information will improve your chances of getting the right shoe for your feet.

■ **Get your feet measured.** Your size can change over time, and footwear that's too small can set you up for an array of problems. Make sure you have a thumb's width of room in front of the end of your big toe while you're standing rather than sitting.

■ **Replace your shoes every 300 to 500 miles.** That's about every 5 to 8 months if you're walking about 3 miles 5 days a week. By the time a walking shoe looks wrecked on the outside, the inside support and cushioning are long gone. I know, it's hard to part with a comfortable pair of old trainers, but you'll be doing yourself and your feet a favour. Worn-out shoes are a common cause of foot, knee and even back pain.

YOUR SOCKS

■ **Look for synthetic fabrics that wick moisture away,** keeping your feet dry and making them less prone to blisters. Avoid all-cotton socks. Since some socks are thick and others are thin, wear your walking socks when you try shoes on because they can affect the fit.

The Metabolism Boost: Muscle in on Belly Fat

I'VE ALWAYS BEEN devoted to strength training. (My daughters know that when I leave for the gym, 'Mummy's going to make muscles.') It gives me confidence and a sense of empowerment. Plus, I just like the way it makes my body feel: toned, strong and healthy. I also know how important it is as I get older. Strength training preserves and even rebuilds precious muscle – the body's calorie-burning engine that fuels metabolism. Beginning as early as in your thirties, you start to lose about ½lb of muscle a year. If you don't take action, that loss can double by the time you hit the menopause. With every pound of muscle lost, your body burns fewer calories, which explains why gaining weight gets easier and losing it gets tougher as you get older. Decreasing muscle mass also makes you weaker, and everyday tasks such as getting out of a chair and climbing the stairs become more difficult. As a result, you start to move less – further contributing to muscle loss and fat gain.

When you challenge a muscle, you create microscopic tears in the muscle tissue. (I know the word *tear* doesn't sound all that healthy, but trust me, in this case it is.) Your body then comes to the rescue and fills those crevices with protein, creating new muscle tissue. This is why you should wait a day between strength-training workouts – to give the muscles time to repair themselves.

Replacing the tissue creates stronger muscles – the result you want, because stronger muscle mass makes our bodies look firmer, tighter and more toned. Most importantly, though, because muscle mass burns about 7 times more calories than fat (about 15 more a day per pound), the more muscle you have, the faster you'll burn calories and lose belly fat.

Strength training increases your energy as well, which makes almost every task easier, so you're more likely to remain active throughout the day.

Finally, strong muscles also protect and build strong bones, which is essential, particularly for a woman. As if losing muscle mass weren't bad enough, women start to lose bone in their mid-thirties as well, a loss that accelerates as they age and gathers even more speed going into the menopause. At that point, some women begin to lose up to 20 per cent of their bone within the first 5 years. Bone loss can lead to accidental breaks and spontaneous fractures (when bones break for no apparent reason), both of which become harder to heal as we get older, as there is less bone to knit the fracture together. Bone loss also leads to spinal curvature, which, in addition to being uncomfortable, makes standing straight impossible and ultimately causes the belly to protrude. Strength training stresses your bones by stretching and pulling muscles and tendons to increase bone density and reduce the risk of osteoporosis. If you already have osteoporosis, strength training can lessen its impact – but check with your doctor before starting any exercise programme.

Here are six other ways in which strength training can improve your health.

■ You'll sleep better. People who strength train regularly are less likely to struggle with insomnia.

■ You'll increase muscle. Each pound burns an extra 15 calories per day.

Ensure Your Safety Outside

- Walk with a friend.
- Choose routes you're familiar with.
- Wear reflective clothing and carry a torch in the dark and at dawn and dusk. Wear bright colours during the day.
- Try to avoid rush hour to reduce your exposure to carbon monoxide.

- Don't carry valuables with you.
- Walk facing traffic so you can see cars coming.
- Carry a mobile phone and ID.
- If you listen to music, keep the volume low enough so you can hear if a car or person is approaching you.

■ You'll improve your balance by strengthening ligaments and tendons.

■ You'll have more stamina. As you grow stronger, you won't fatigue as easily.

■ You'll reduce your diabetes risk. Lean muscle tissue helps your body metabolize blood sugar.

■ You'll minimize the appearance of cellulite. Building firm, compact muscle will smooth out lumpy lower-body fat.

Before You Start: Strength-Training Basics

IF YOU'RE NOT yet doing any strength training, *now is the time to start!* If you're currently lifting weights, then try ramping it up a notch.

■ THE TERMS: If you're picking up dumbbells for the first time, here are some strength-training basics. The word *rep* is short for *repetition*: for example, each time you lift and lower a dumbbell, or roll your upper body off the floor and then lower it back down, it's considered one repetition. A specific number of reps (8, 10, 12 and so on) is called a *set*.

■ YOUR WEIGHTS: Many women train with weights too light to produce the metabolic boost and body firming they want. Don't be afraid of heavier weights – you won't get big, bulky muscles (women simply don't have enough of the hormones needed for those types of results), but you will get stronger and firmer faster. For the best results, the weight you choose should be heavy enough that by your last rep, you feel like you can't do any more using good form. If you can, you need to increase the amount of weight you're lifting. If you can't do at least eight reps, then the weight is too heavy: choose a lighter weight or try the easier version of the exercise. Because some muscles are bigger than others, you'll need to use heavier weights for exercises that target your chest, back, legs and buttocks. For smaller muscles like your arms and shoulders, you'll probably want lighter weights.

■ YOUR ROUTINE: In The Metabolism Boost, you'll begin with one set of 10 reps and progress to two sets of 15 reps during the 4-week programme. Remember, if at any point the weight you're lifting isn't fatiguing the targeted muscles by your last rep, it's time to increase the amount of weight you're using or try the harder variation. (For the ab exercises, you can try the harder version or increase your number of reps.)

■ YOUR EQUIPMENT: You will need two sets of dumbbells for this section of the programme – light and heavy. If you are a beginner, try starting with a 3-lb and a 5-lb set. If you're more experienced, a 5-lb and 8-lb set is a good place to begin. Remember, these are general guidelines, so adjust the amount of weight you're lifting, based on my recommendations above. It's easy to determine your correct weight: if the set is so easy that you feel at the end that you can keep going, you're probably not working hard enough – that is, you're not doing enough reps or the weights are too light. If, on the other hand, you can barely get the last rep in for the last set, then your choice of weight and reps is just right. Eventually, as your muscles get stronger, you'll become accustomed to the number of sets and reps you're doing. That's the time to move on.

What time should I exercise?

A: Some surveys have shown that morning exercisers are more consistent because there are fewer opportunities to get sidetracked and skip it than with an evening workout. But if you're not a morning person, the snooze button may be all you need to distract you. The most important consideration should be finding a time when you're most willing and able to exercise. Fit your workouts into your life when it's most convenient for you – otherwise, other activities will always bump exercise off your schedule. There's no significant impact on the calories you burn or how quickly you'll see results based on the time of day you exercise. What matters most is that you *just do it.*

In **The Belly Routine**, we give you a specific number of reps to follow, but you can select from our suggestions for how to make it easier or harder, depending on what works best for you. Just remember that if you want to develop lean muscle tissue, you must select a weight that's challenging.

THE METABOLISM BOOST WEEKLY PLAN

WEEK	DAY 2	DAY 4	DAY 6
1	10 reps	10 reps	10 reps
2	15 reps	15 reps	15 reps
3	2 sets, 10 reps	2 sets, 10 reps	2 sets, 10 reps
4	2 sets, 15 reps	2 sets, 15 reps	2 sets, 15 reps

Lunge Press

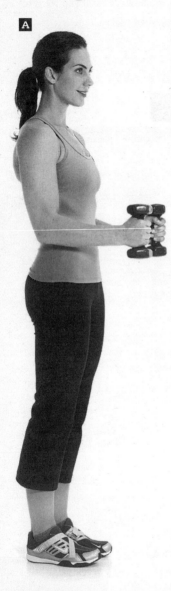

A

A. Stand with feet together. Holding a dumbbell in each hand, bend arms to 90 degrees so dumbbells are in front of you, forearms parallel to floor, palms facing each other.

B. Step right foot 60cm to 1m (2 to 3ft) behind you, landing on ball of foot. Bend knees, lowering right knee towards floor until left thigh is parallel to floor. Keep left knee directly over ankle. At the same time, press dumbbells behind you, straightening arms. Hold for a second, then press into left foot, standing back up, bringing feet together, and bending arms back to start position. Do 1 set, then repeat with opposite leg.

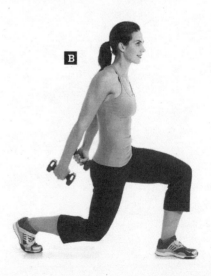

B

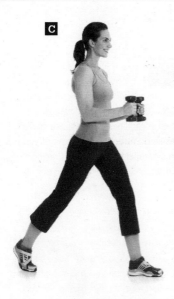

MAKE IT EASIER

C. Do standing lunges by starting with left foot 60cm to 1m (2 to 3ft) in front of right foot, right heel off floor. Maintain this position for 1 set, then switch legs and repeat.

MAKE IT HARDER

D. As you stand back up from the lunge position, raise right knee in front of you to hip height, leg bent 90 degrees. At the same time, bend arms back to start position. Hold for 1 second, balancing on left foot, then swing right foot behind you and repeat. Complete 1 set, and then repeat with opposite leg.

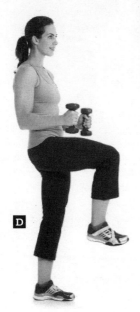

Squat Curl

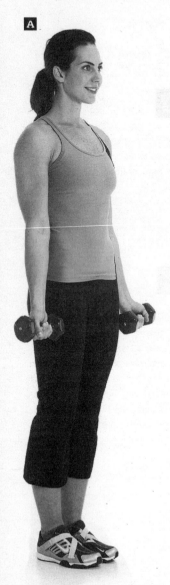

A

**MAIN
MOVE**

A. Stand with feet together, holding a dumbbell in each hand, arms down at sides, palms facing forwards.

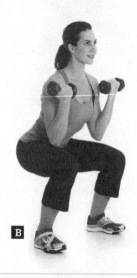

B

B. Step right foot about 60cm (2ft) out to side and bend knees and hips as if you were sitting back into a chair. Sit back as far as possible, keeping knees behind toes. At the same time, bend elbows, curling dumbbells up towards shoulders. Don't move upper arms or shoulders. As you stand back up, bring feet together and lower dumbbells. Complete 1 set, and then repeat, stepping to side with left foot.

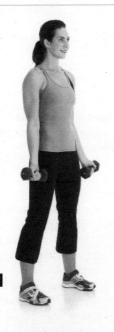

MAKE IT EASIER

C. Start with feet about shoulder-width apart and maintain this position as you do squats, without stepping to the side.

C

MAKE IT HARDER

D. As you stand back up from the squat position, raise left knee, bringing it in front of you to hip height, leg bent 90 degrees. Hold for 1 second, balancing on right foot, then swing left foot out to side and repeat. Complete 1 set, then repeat with opposite leg.

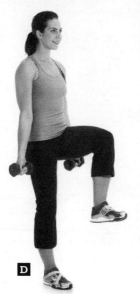

D

Side Lunge & Raise

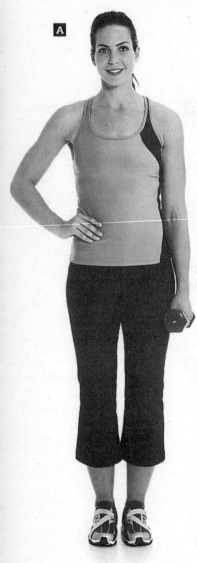

A

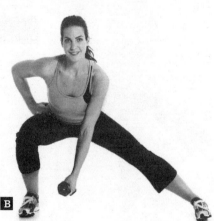

B

MAIN MOVE

A. Stand with feet together and hold a dumbbell in left hand with arm at side, palm facing in. Place right hand on hip.

B. Step right foot 60cm to 1m (2 to 3ft) out to side and bend right knee into a lunge, sitting back and bringing dumbbell towards right ankle. Keep right knee behind toes. Press off right foot and stand back up, bringing feet together. From this position, raise left arm out to left side until it's at shoulder height, and lift right leg out to opposite side, as high as possible (like photo opposite, below). Hold for a second, then return to start position. Complete 1 set, then switch sides and repeat.

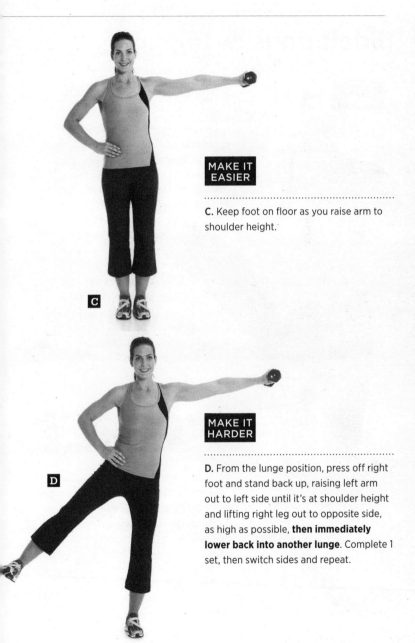

MAKE IT EASIER

....

C. Keep foot on floor as you raise arm to shoulder height.

MAKE IT HARDER

....

D. From the lunge position, press off right foot and stand back up, raising left arm out to left side until it's at shoulder height and lifting right leg out to opposite side, as high as possible, **then immediately lower back into another lunge**. Complete 1 set, then switch sides and repeat.

Push-up Row

MAIN MOVE

A. Holding a dumbbell in each hand, get down on hands and knees. Walk hands forwards so body forms a straight line from head to knees, and hands are directly beneath shoulders and feet are in the air.

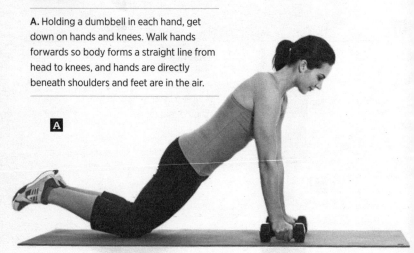

A

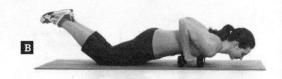

B

B. Bend elbows out to sides, lowering chest almost to floor. Press into hands, straightening arms back to start position. **C.** Then bend right elbow back, pulling dumbbell towards chest, keeping arm close to body. Lower dumbbell back to floor, and repeat from beginning, this time doing a row with left arm. Continue alternating rows for a full set, doing an extra rep each time so you do an equal number of rows with each arm.

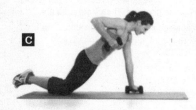

C

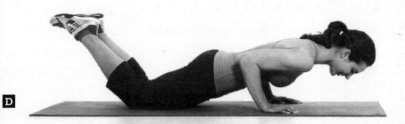

D

MAKE IT EASIER

Break up the moves. Do one set of push-ups without dumbbells. **D.** Then get on hands and knees and do a set of rows with each arm.

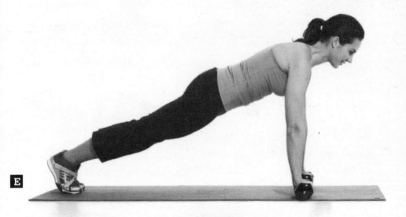

E

MAKE IT HARDER

E. Do full push-ups, balancing on hands and toes.

The Belly Routine: Carve Those Abs

PART 3 OF the Flat Belly Workout focuses, of course, on your ab muscles. But I have another confession to make: when I was younger, I often skipped those last 5 minutes of my step class that were devoted to ab exercises for one reason: they consisted solely of crunches. *Bo-ring.* Plus they never seemed to do much for my middle. Our belly-toning workout is a combined routine that includes Pilates, traditional ab moves and balance exercises to ensure that you're toning your mid-section from every angle. All of these moves have been lab-tested and are guaranteed to deliver better results than ordinary crunches.

The roll-up works the main belly muscle, the rectus abdominis, which runs from the bottom of your ribs down to your pelvis, and is 80 per cent more effective than a standard crunch.

The bicycle move is our choice if you only have time for one exercise. It targets the main ab muscle more effectively while also working your obliques, the muscles that wrap around your torso. This generates 190 per cent more activity than when you do a simple crunch, according to an American study.

Moves like the plank and arm and leg extension work both your abdominal and back muscles at the same time. Strong back muscles allow you to

Stretch Your Workout Benefits

The most important thing you can do before exercise is to warm up with gentle activity. The best time to stretch is post-workout, when your muscles are warm and pliable. Stretching then also helps promote recovery and will improve your posture so you stand taller, making your belly look flatter instantly.

These three stretches target the major muscle groups that you'll be working. Gently ease in and out of the stretches,

holding each for 10 seconds. Don't bounce. Do each stretch 3 to 6 times, taking deep breaths throughout.

■ QUAD STRETCH Standing with feet together, bend left leg behind you, bringing that foot towards buttocks. (You can hold on to a chair or wall with right hand for balance if needed.) Grasp left foot with left hand and tuck hips under so you feel a stretch in the front of left thigh

stand taller, improving posture – bonus – and helping your belly look flatter almost instantly.

Finally, the pike zeros in on those lower abs. Since the rectus abdominis is one long, continuous muscle, you can't completely isolate your upper and lower abs. But this exercise allows you to maximize the amount of work that the muscle fibres in the lower portion of that muscle are doing, activating it more than regular crunches, while also stimulating the upper portion.

Bottom line? Not a crunch in the bunch. And now you know why.

THE BELLY ROUTINE WEEKLY PLAN

WEEK	DAY 1	DAY 3	DAY 5
1	10 reps	10 reps	10 reps
2	15 reps	15 reps	15 reps
3	2 sets, 10 reps	2 sets, 10 reps	2 sets, 10 reps
4	2 sets, 15 reps	2 sets, 15 reps	2 sets, 15 reps

and hip. Hold for 10 seconds and release. Switch legs and repeat.

■ CALF STRETCH Stand with right foot about 60cm to 1m (2 to 3ft) in front of left, toes pointing forwards. Place hands on right thigh and bend right knee, keeping left leg straight and pressing left heel into floor so you feel a stretch in left calf. Hold for 10 seconds and release. Switch legs and repeat.

■ HAMSTRING STRETCH From the calf stretch position, step back foot in 15 to 30cm (6 to 12in). Straighten front leg, lifting front toes off floor, and bend back leg and sit back, placing hands on thigh. It is very important not to lock your front knee. You should feel a stretch down the back of the thigh of your straight leg. Hold for 10 seconds and release. Switch legs and repeat.

Bicycle

A. Lie face-up with knees above hips, calves parallel to floor and hands behind head.

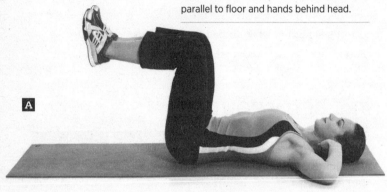

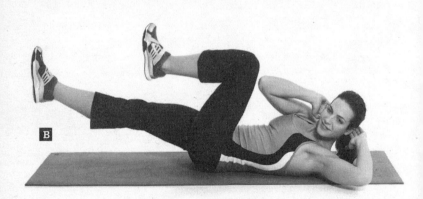

B. Contract abs, raising head and shoulders off floor as you extend right leg so it's about 25cm (10in) off floor. Twist to left, bringing right elbow and left knee towards each other. Don't pull on your neck; the work should come from your abs. Hold for a second, then switch sides, twisting to right. That's 1 rep.

· ·

C. Keep feet flat on floor with knees bent
as you lift and twist upper body.

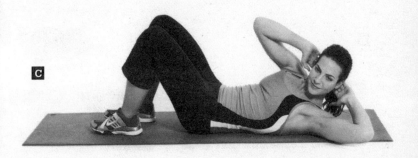

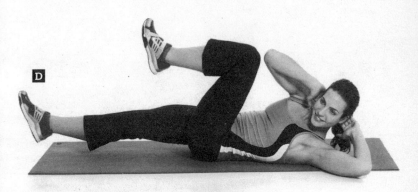

· ·

D. Lower extended leg further so it's about
8cm (3in) off floor.

Hover

A. Lie face down with upper body propped on forearms and elbows directly beneath shoulders. Toes are tucked.

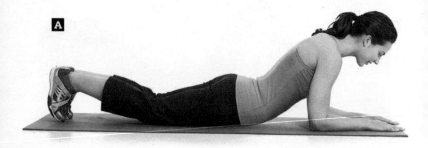

A

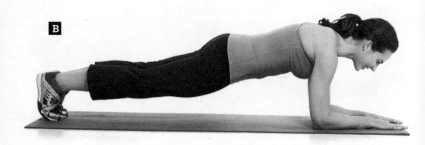

B

B. Contract torso muscles, lifting belly and legs off floor so body forms a straight line from head to heels. Keep abs tight so belly doesn't droop. Hold for 15 seconds (increase by 15 seconds each week so that by week 4 you're holding for 1 minute). One rep is all you need to do.

C. Keep knees on floor and just lift belly, balancing on knees and forearms. Stay in this position.

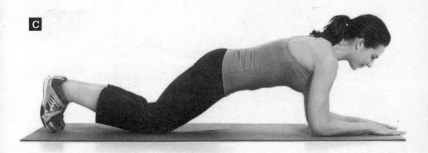

C

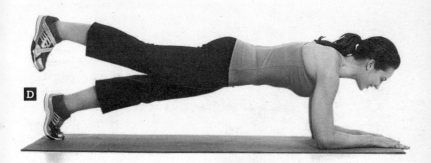

D

D. Raise right foot off floor and hold for half the time, then switch legs and hold for remaining time.

Roll-Up

MAIN MOVE

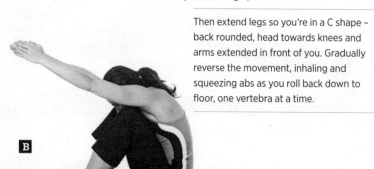

A. Lie on back with arms extended over-head and legs bent, feet flat on floor.

B. Inhale and raise arms over chest. Then exhale and roll head towards chest, lifting head and shoulders off floor. (Keep arms next to ears throughout the move.) Press inner thighs together and pull navel in towards spine. Slowly peel off floor until you're sitting up.

Then extend legs so you're in a C shape – back rounded, head towards knees and arms extended in front of you. Gradually reverse the movement, inhaling and squeezing abs as you roll back down to floor, one vertebra at a time.

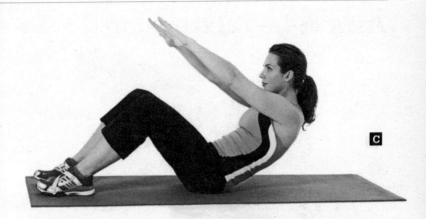

MAKE IT EASIER

C. Sit upright on floor with knees bent, feet flat and arms extended at shoulder height in front of you. As you exhale, roll back only about 45 degrees, one vertebra at a time, keeping abs tight. Then roll back up.

MAKE IT HARDER

D. Do the move with legs extended the whole time.

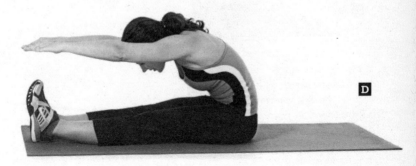

Arm & Leg Extension

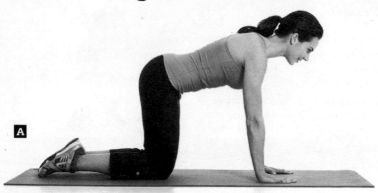

MAIN MOVE

A. Kneel with hands directly beneath shoulders, and knees directly beneath hips.

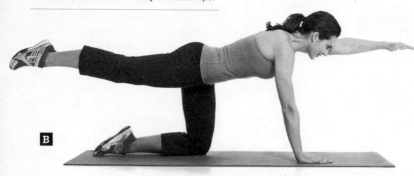

B. Keeping back straight and head in line with spine, simultaneously raise left arm and right leg, extending them in line with back so fingers are pointing straight ahead and toes are pointing behind you. Hold for a second, then lower. Perform 1 set, then switch arms and legs and repeat.

....

C. Instead of lifting and lowering arm and leg, hold them in line with back for 15 seconds, then repeat on opposite side. One rep on each side is enough. Increase the amount of time you hold the move until you can do it for a full minute.

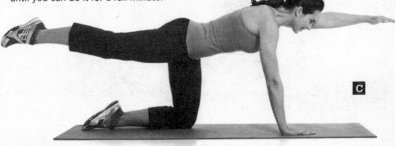

C

....

D. When arm and leg are raised, contract abs and draw left elbow and right knee together beneath torso, holding for a second. Extend and repeat. Perform 1 set, then switch arms and legs and repeat.

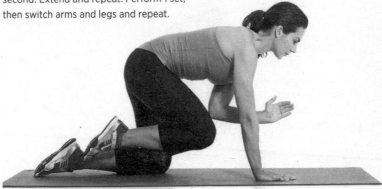

Ab Pike

MAIN MOVE

A. Lie face-up with arms at sides. Bend legs so feet are off floor, thighs over hips.

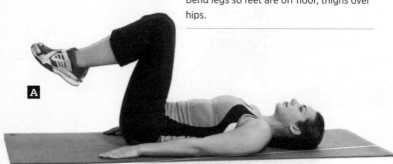

A

B. As you pull abs towards spine, lift hips up off floor, keeping legs bent. Keep hands and arms relaxed so you don't use them to help lift. Hold for a second, then slowly lower hips to floor and bend legs.

B

C. Lie with legs bent, feet flat on floor. Contract abs, pressing small of back into floor and curl hips up, doing a pelvic tilt, without lifting feet.

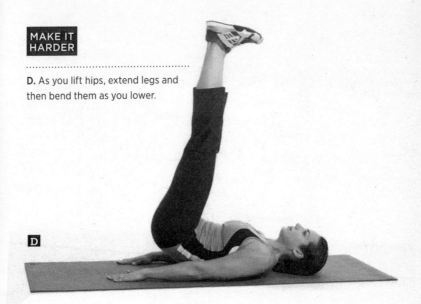

C

D. As you lift hips, extend legs and then bend them as you lower.

D

PUTTING IT ALL TOGETHER: YOUR 28-DAY FLAT BELLY WORKOUT PLAN

WEEK	DAY 1	DAY 2	DAY 3
1	Fat Blast Walk 30 min	Calorie Torch Walk 25 min	Fat Blast Walk 30 min
	The Belly Routine 10 reps	The Metabolism Boost 10 reps	The Belly Routine 10 reps
2	Fat Blast Walk 45 min	Calorie Torch Walk 35 min	Fat Blast Walk 45 min
	The Belly Routine 15 reps	The Metabolism Boost 15 reps	The Belly Routine 15 reps
3	Fat Blast Walk 60 min	Calorie Torch Walk 45 min	Fat Blast Walk 60 min
	The Belly Routine 2 sets, 10 reps	The Metabolism Boost 2 sets, 10 reps	The Belly Routine 2 sets, 10 reps
4	Fat Blast Walk 60 min	Calorie Torch Walk 45 min	Fat Blast Walk 60 min
	The Belly Routine 2 sets, 15 reps	The Metabolism Boost 2 sets, 15 reps	The Belly Routine 2 sets, 15 reps

DAY 4	DAY 5	DAY 6	DAY 7
Calorie Torch Walk 25 min	Fat Blast Walk 30 min	Calorie Torch Walk 25 min	
The Metabolism Boost 10 reps	The Belly Routine 10 reps	The Metabolism Boost 10 reps	REST
Calorie Torch Walk 35 min	Fat Blast Walk 45 min	Calorie Torch Walk 35 min	
The Metabolism Boost 15 reps	The Belly Routine 15 reps	The Metabolism Boost 15 reps	REST
Calorie Torch Walk 45 min	Fat Blast Walk 60 min	Calorie Torch Walk 45 min	
The Metabolism Boost 2 sets, 10 reps	The Belly Routine 2 sets, 10 reps	The Metabolism Boost 2 sets, 10 reps	REST
Calorie Torch Walk 45 min	Fat Blast Walk 60 min	Calorie Torch Walk 45 min	
The Metabolism Boost 2 sets, 15 reps	The Belly Routine 2 sets, 15 reps	The Metabolism Boost 2 sets, 15 reps	REST

Staying Motivated

AND NOW, A word about attitude. By now, you get it. Believing in yourself is integral to this entire Flat Belly journey. I see the power of attitude at first-hand in every weight loss success story I hear and every time I meet someone who's faced a life challenge head-on. The right outlook and perspective is what I always call the 'special sauce'. It means better results, faster results, and results that last.

I urge you to keep this in mind when the going gets rough: changing your thought process can change your whole workout experience. In fact, your mind is so powerful that it can strengthen muscles without lifting a single dumbbell. When researchers at the Cleveland Clinic in the US got healthy volunteers to imagine that they were contracting the muscles in their hands, they increased hand strength by 35 per cent. While this field of study is just beginning, imagine what your mind can do during an actual workout.

4 Reasons to Work Out to Music

1. You'll feel happier. A groundbreaking brain-imaging study from McGill University in Canada showed for the first time that music activates the same reward or pleasure centres in the brain that respond to the good feelings associated with eating and – believe it or not – sex.[5]

2. You'll move faster. Australian researchers discovered that the faster the beat, the more vigorously you work out. Other research has shown that exercisers who listen to music have more endurance and thus exercise longer, burning more calories.

3. You'll get cleverer. In the first study to look at the combined effects of music and exercise on mental performance, Charles Emery, the study's leading author and a professor of psychology at Ohio State University in the US, found that this duo increased scores on a verbal fluency test.[6]

4. You'll lose belly fat faster. Women who exercised to music lost as much as 8lb more than women who broke a sweat in silence.

Now, armed with this information, head into every workout imagining yourself strong, energized and light as a feather. Don't recall moments from your tough day or dwell on how tired you feel. Instead, imagine yourself walking on clouds or that an invisible force is lifting you up, helping you take that next step, lift that weight or complete that move. Your mind is a powerful thing. Use it! If you take just a few seconds to adjust your attitude, you won't believe how much easier, faster and enjoyable your workout will be.

What if I'm an avid exerciser? Should I stick with my regular routine or do this one?

If you have an exercise programme you love, absolutely keep it up. You're more likely to stick with exercise if you're doing something you enjoy. But I would encourage you to compare your workouts to those recommended here, and maybe make some minor adjustments to your exercise plan to maximize its belly-flattening potential. Here are some questions to ask yourself as you review your plan.

■ *Am I lifting weights at least 2 days a week?*
If not, consider adding **The Metabolism Boost** moves on pages 250 to 257 to your workout schedule. If you are but want to see better results, aim for 3 days a week of strength training, working in some of the combined moves from **The Metabolism Boost**. By working multiple body parts at the same time, you'll burn more calories.

■ *Am I doing 30 to 60 minutes of cardio exercise (walking, biking, jogging, swimming, using a cardio machine like an elliptical or stairclimber) at least 5 days a week?*
If not, increase the length or frequency of your workouts to boost your daily calorie burn. If you are but want to see better results, turn three of your sessions into interval workouts – like the **Calorie Torch** walk. Or, turn any cardio activity into an interval routine by increasing the intensity for 30 to 60 seconds and then slowing down to your usual pace for 2 to 5 minutes.

■ *Am I doing any belly-focused exercises at least 2 days a week?*
If not, start by just doing one or two moves from **The Belly Routine** on pages 260 to 269 per session to firm up your mid-section.

READ A FLAT BELLY
SUCCESS
STORY

Evelyn Gomer

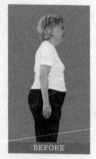

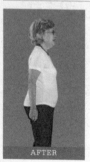

POUNDS LOST:

6

IN 32 DAYS

ALL-OVER INCHES LOST:

8.5

EVELYN GOMER'S MOTIVATION TO TRY THE *FLAT BELLY DIET* came from her friends – indirectly, anyway. 'For years, I was a city person. Most city women are skinny and dress beautifully, and that was me for years – until I moved away from the city.' As Evelyn tells it, 'I married late in life and moved to the suburbs, where the women were more, well, matronly. So for whatever reason, I just let myself go – completely.' She and her husband moved back to the city centre, and she found her city friends were still skinny and svelte – but she wasn't. 'I wanted to get back into that,' she says. 'So when I heard about this diet, I jumped at the chance to try it.' It's not that she hadn't dieted before. She had – but not with any lasting success. 'This one? What a blessing!'

The first really wonderful thing she found was that she was never hungry. 'I'm very uncomfortable when I'm hungry. My stomach growls, and I get very tired and listless. But eating the four meals a day worked for me. And those MUFAs!' Like most of the Flat Belly dieters, Evelyn had never heard of a MUFA before being introduced to the diet, so when she heard she could have nuts, she was happier than happy. 'I adore nuts – all kinds. They actually helped alleviate any yen for richer desserts. I still can't believe that something so fattening can be so healthy,' she says. 'I travel with a jar of peanut butter just in case I'm not in a place where I can find what I want to eat. I can be satisfied just nibbling on nuts. But there are so many other wonderful things to choose from, too.'

Evelyn is all about convenience. She read the 28 days of meals and recipes and selected about 20 meals that she could be happy with and that didn't require '50 million ingredients'. She's been making those same meals over and over. She says that after a while you get to know them by heart and you don't have to read what you need. You do a major shop, and you have all the ingredients in the house.

She brings up a further benefit she has seen from the *Flat Belly Diet,* one in addition to the weight she lost over 4 weeks. It seems her husband is getting thinner, too. 'No,' she says, 'he's not on the diet. It's just that I haven't been cooking much, so he's fending for himself and eating a lot less than he usually eats. He's lost weight, and he's very happy about that.'

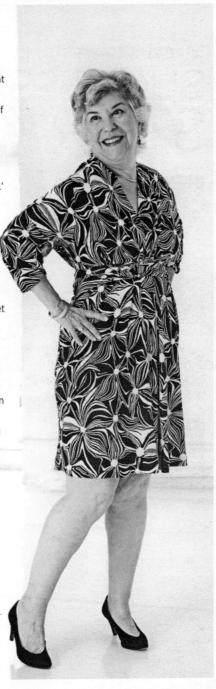

10

YOUR GUIDE TO
DAY 33
AND BEYOND

HERE ARE TWO revealing statistics: on the one hand, a recent US survey found that the percentage of people dieting to lose weight at any given time has fallen to 29 per cent, down from 33 per cent in 2004.[1] Yet, on the other hand, people are beginning to eat more healthily in growing, even stunning, numbers. Fifty-seven per cent of shoppers are trying to eat more healthily, up from 45 per cent in 2000.[2]

Westerners are eating more fruits and vegetables and whole grains than in the past, and in some surveys as many as 90 per cent are doing something to improve the healthiness of their meals, like limiting salt, sugar or saturated fat or paying more attention to portions. That says to me that people are more interested in making food choices that impact on their long-term health than they are in following some gimmicky, quick-fix plan. That's why I wanted the *Flat Belly Diet* to be – first and foremost – something readers could sustain for the rest of their lives.

So, here we are. You've presumably finished the first 32 days of the *Flat Belly Diet*, so let's take a look back at what you've achieved. If you've followed the parameters of this plan (eating your MUFAs at every meal, limiting calories to 1,600 a day, exercising on a regular basis in a sensible, efficient way and coming to a deeper realization about how you think about food), then you've taken the first and most difficult step towards a healthier future. And – a nice bonus here – you've probably lost some of the deadliest fat you can have: belly fat.

I also hope you've learned a few things that will make living the *Flat Belly Diet* lifestyle even more rewarding. You know the anatomy and physiology of the digestive system better than ever before. You understand why the fat you can't see is sometimes scarier than the fat that pokes out over your jeans. And you've read about the intricate connection between stress, cortisol and your body. Putting all this knowledge to work for you, your belly and your health in an ongoing way is as simple as permanently adopting the three *Flat Belly Diet* rules that are probably quite familiar to you by now. I hope you've discovered that it really is possible to follow the *Flat Belly Diet* for ever.

Our test panellists certainly did. After ending the test phase of the *Flat Belly Diet*, every single one, without being asked, said they planned to stick to the programme. Why? Because they lost weight and reduced their measurements and never felt deprived. Because week after week they reported no hunger, energy through the roof and no cravings. They gave the meals and recipes rave reviews. And they loved knowing that once they understood the plan, they didn't have to count the days until they could eat satisfying meals again.

Remember, succeeding on the *Flat Belly Diet* promises an even greater reward than a visually attractive silhouette: it promises a longer, healthier life. This chapter is all about getting you fully armed to reap *all* the rewards of the *Flat Belly Diet* – flat belly included – for decades to come.

Flat Belly for Life: Rules to Eat By

▓ **Rule #1** Stick to 400 calories per meal.

▓ **Rule #2** Never go more than 4 hours without eating.

▓ **Rule #3** Eat a MUFA at every meal.

RULE #1: STICK TO 400 CALORIES PER MEAL

I'M NOT GOING to mince words here: to keep your weight down and your metabolism on track, you must continue to control your daily calorie intake – that is, stick to about 400 calories per meal, 1,600 per day. Why, you're wondering, do you have to maintain the same daily calorie intake that got you to your goal, *after* you've reached it? Because the fact of the matter is, 1,600 calories is enough to keep up your energy, support your immune system and maintain your precious calorie-burning muscle (so you won't feel run-down, moody or hungry), but it's not enough calories to allow you to gain back your belly fat (and make you more vulnerable to all the attendant health risks).

I am in no way sentencing you to a life of deprivation or boredom here. You've been eating the *Flat Belly Diet* way for 32 days, and you know at first-hand how satisfying and hunger-free this lifestyle is. One of the main reasons the *Flat Belly Diet* worked for you is that the food is nothing less than fabulous. And there's no shortage of it. And boredom? Forget about it. Between the quick-fix meals, Snack Packs and recipes, as well as a multitude of approved packaged and fast food items, you have hundreds of choices, whether or not you have the time (or the inclination) to cook.

RULE #2: NEVER GO MORE THAN 4 HOURS WITHOUT EATING

THIS IS YOUR tried-and-true routine by now. You've established a rhythm, and your body has responded – by becoming accustomed to having three MUFA-rich 400-calorie meals at 4-hour intervals, as well as a healthy Snack Pack at whatever time of day suits you. You now know how it feels to keep your energy up, your blood sugar steady, your metabolism revved – what it's like to have control of your appetite. And you've seen the results, belly-wise. Stick with it and it will continue to benefit your health and your waistline.

RULE #3: EAT A MUFA AT EVERY MEAL

OVER THE PAST few weeks, you have come to know MUFAs well (and love them as dearly as I do, I'm sure!), those little miracle workers in your belly that help you feel full *and* lose visceral fat from your middle. You've also discovered how easy – and tasty – it is to include small amounts of these healthy fats in your meals. Even if you can't work in a MUFA at every single meal you ever eat, you know that they are found mainly in vegetable oils, nuts, seeds, olives and avocados. They are about as easy to come by as they are to love, and it won't be difficult for you to put the MUFA rule into practice most of the time. And if you don't know the MUFA list by heart at this point, you can always turn to page 101 for a quick reference.

A Flat Belly for Life: Strategies to Live By

TIME AND AGAIN throughout this book I've told you, the *Flat Belly Diet* is about *attitude*. Well, guess what – so is your healthy, flat-bellied future.

I've supplied you with tools and tricks galore that, as you move forward beyond Day 32, are going to be no less important to nourishing and fortifying you than the Flat Belly meals and MUFAs. These tools and tricks have been as integral to your success as the foods you've eaten. You've used them to make major changes. And they'll be just as essential to your ongoing health and well-being.

I've boiled it down to a few key practices and pointers. Use these as a guide in your journey ahead.

KEEPING A JOURNAL

As ALREADY NOTED, keeping a journal is probably the single most important thing you can do going forward to help you maintain your focus on your long-term health goals. Trust me when I say it will help you stay on track. I'm not suggesting that you write something for 15 minutes every day

The Danger of Skipping Meals

It doesn't pay to try to dip below the 1,600-calories-a-day mark. Believe me, I understand the temptation. We've all been led to believe that the fewer calories we ingest, the faster we'll lose weight. But weight loss isn't quite that simple. If you drastically cut down on the amount of food you eat for any extended period of time, your body's natural response is to slow things down in order to conserve fat. For those of us who aspire to flatter bellies, that 'starvation response' is the last thing we need.

Here's what happens: if you take in too few calories, your body starts breaking down muscle tissue to use for fuel. That muscle loss can drastically affect your metabolism, often for long periods of time. The reason is simple: muscle is metabolically active tissue

that requires a certain number of calories each day to maintain itself, whether or not it's in use. So the more muscle you have, the more calories you burn. As your muscle mass drops, so does your body's need for calories to sustain it. Let's say a dieter on a too-strict plan loses 15lb – 10lb of which is fat and 5lb of which is muscle. Let's also assume that every pound of muscle burns about 50 calories a day. With this muscle tissue gone, the dieter must now consume 250 (5 times 50) fewer calories a day in order to *maintain* her 15lb weight loss.

Of course, most dieters don't stick to the strict routine for long; they return to their pre-diet eating habits. And that's what puts them at risk of regaining all their lost weight – and then some more.

for the rest of your life. I am, however, urging you to keep a journal in your repertoire of health tools. Just as no parent should be without a thermometer in the medicine cabinet, I firmly believe that no woman should be without the means to record her thoughts and feelings on paper (or on a computer). Your journal is your emotional thermometer. Your thoughts are the clues to all your destructive insecurities and all your inner power. Why on earth would you consider ignoring them?

SASS FROM SASS

'Avoid These Common Pitfalls'

As a dietitian, I've helped hundreds of people lose weight, but I've also lived with a successful 'loser' for over a decade. Seeing my husband, Jack, lose more than 3½stone (50lb) and never put it back on has shown me at first-hand that, while it's not always easy, it is possible to lose a significant amount of weight *and* keep it off. A recent study looked at the key reasons why successful losers so often regain the weight they've lost. I can say that Jack's a pro at avoiding each one of these pitfalls, and you can be, too.

Pitfall #1: failing to plan in advance before social situations. Prevent it by bringing your own meals or snacks when you're going out with friends or family, or host get-togethers at your house so you have more control over the menu.

Pitfall #2: feeling deprived. According to our testers, this wasn't an issue on the *Flat Belly Diet*. Over and over again we heard that they didn't feel deprived at all and even felt a little guilty about how full and satisfied they were. That's because the food on this plan is delicious and includes healthy indulgences like chocolate, nuts, cheese and berries.

Pitfall #3: underestimating the number of calories in foods. We've made this one a no-brainer. The *Flat Belly Diet* controls your calories for you so you can't go overboard.
                                                  – Cynthia

STAY MINDFUL

WHENEVER YOU NEED a quick attitude adjustment from frantic to focused, call on the Mind Tricks from Chapter 5. They're fast – just minutes apiece – but extremely effective at jolting you out of a stress-fuelled stupor and adjusting your emotional relationship to eating. They'll help you slow down, take your time and savour your meals, so you won't be tempted to overindulge or eat too quickly.

MANAGE STRESS

THE STRESS–BELLY FAT connection is clear. Manage stress and you are one step closer to managing your belly fat for ever. Writing in your journal can be a great stress reliever, but so can daily exercise. (Another reason that I like to walk to and from work is that I get to work out solutions to office crises in my head, entertaining passers-by by occasionally talking to myself.) If you need more ideas to help get your stress under control, periodically revisit the stress-busting strategies in Chapter 4 and use them as a checklist.

GATHER A SUPPORT TEAM

ONE OF THE best ways to stay on track and stay motivated is to have a support team behind you. Regardless of how motivated you are, long-term success is always easier with help from others. Even one person will do – just someone to tell you you're doing really well every once in a while. Having people in your life who understand and accept your dreams can make all the difference in the world. Your supporters don't have to be members of your family or even good friends, so long as they respect your goals.

Results in the Real World

SCALES NOT BUDGING? At a certain point, every dieter hits a plateau. Here's why it happens. The *Flat Belly Diet* is designed only to give you enough calories – 1,600 – to support a healthy, 'ideal' weight. If you weigh more than your ideal weight, you are consuming more than 1,600 calories a day. You may jump up and down and tell me that no, you know for a fact that you're only eating 1,200 calories a day, you're starving, and you still don't lose weight. And I would say *Not true!* Just as you need a certain amount of wood to heat a log cabin, you need a certain amount of calories to keep yourself alive. And the more you weigh, the more calories you need to maintain that weight. Just by going on this plan, you've created a calorie deficit that will allow you to drop pounds. With every pound you lose, however, this calorie deficit shrinks, so as you get closer and closer to your weight goal, it takes longer and longer to lose the next pound.

It doesn't seem fair, but it's the laws of physics! On this plan, you should never hit a true plateau (that is, no net loss). But at times it might feel like your weight loss has stalled. If you're following the plan – and keeping a food journal – I can assure you it has not stalled. It has just slowed. Think about it like this – if you were losing 2lb a week, then just 1lb a week, you'll eventually get to $\frac{1}{2}$lb a week, then $\frac{1}{4}$lb. Those incremental losses probably won't register on your scales, but a loss is still a loss. Remember that even $\frac{1}{4}$lb of fat loss is half a packet of butter zapped from your body. That's still amazing progress in 1 week!

The *Flat Belly Diet* to Go: The Angst-Free Guide to Dining Out

OK, YOU'VE GOT this gorgeous, flat belly, you're full of energy and you feel absolutely wonderful. Now it's time to celebrate. Maybe it's your anniversary. Or your birthday. Or maybe you're just feeling happy. Dinner out? Why not?

Just remember, you are there to celebrate, not binge. And if you stick to the programme – or even a slightly modified version – you will wake up feeling good, not guilty, tomorrow. Go ahead, treat yourself to something special. If you plan ahead, there's no reason why you shouldn't be able to enjoy a meal anywhere you want, and that includes pizza with your girlfriends after an afternoon of shopping. Following these guidelines will help you stay on track.

■ Eat what you would normally eat throughout the day. Skipping a meal in order to save calories for later just increases the chances that you will overeat at dinner. You can also up your exercise – the added calorie burn will help offset a splurge like dessert.

■ Have a light snack before you go out. Good options include *Flat Belly Diet* smoothies or anything that incudes a MUFA. The MUFA will take the edge off your hunger and help you pass on the bread basket.

■ Be the first at the table to order. This will keep you from being tempted by others' choices.

■ Try to leave some food on your plate. The old 'clean plate' rules from childhood no longer apply.

DID YOU KNOW ?

Research published in the *Journal of the American Medical Association* revealed that women who exercised 5 days per week for 30 to 45 minutes at a time for a full year were able to reduce belly fat by 3 to 6 per cent.[7]

Portion Patrol

PERHAPS THE MOST important tip for dining out is to watch the size of your portions. It goes without saying that anything called 'super size' is something to be avoided, but beware of dishes that don't advertise their generous proportions yet provide enough for two or three people. It always helps to have a visual reference to help moderate your portions of different foods when dining out. For example:

■ One 'serving' of cooked rice or pasta is considered to be 100g (3½oz). This is about the size of half a cricket ball. If you're trying to limit your portion of rice or pasta to two servings: think one cricket ball. Most Chinese restaurants provide far more than this amount of rice.

■ One standard-size slice of bread is considered one 'serving' of bread. Compare rolls, buns and other bread products to this mental image and adjust your portion size accordingly: if the bun for your chicken sandwich or burger looks larger than two slices of bread, leave some bread on the plate.

■ Ninety grams (3oz) of cooked meat, the size of a deck of cards or woman's palm, is considered one 'serving'. Most restaurants provide far more than this amount in a main course. Clever ways to cut back include ordering a half portion, having a sandwich instead of a main course or sharing a meal.

■ A single portion of grated cheese is considered to be 30g (1oz). That's about the size of a golf ball. Healthy adults need two to three servings of milk, yogurt or cheese per day. If cheese is your weakness, think 'golf ball' the next time you sprinkle cheese on your food.

To Finish

I'D LIKE TO finish by reminding you of the very last question I asked you in Chapter 4: *Who are you doing this for?* There is still only one acceptable answer to that question. That answer is '*for me*'.

This plan was created to help you see that focusing on yourself isn't an exercise in selfishness. In this day and age, we are all overly committed to other people, whether it's the attention we lavish on our children and spouse, or the time we spend in our jobs or the effort we put into building our communities. But I speak from experience when I tell you that none of those commitments is worth anything if you aren't first and foremost committed to yourself. The *Flat Belly Diet* is not a vanity ploy. Of course, it's a weight-loss plan designed to give you a sexier waistline. But it's not a crazy detox diet that promises you the abs of a 20-year-old. It is a weight-loss plan based on the most credible – and safe – science that targets the most dangerous type of fat you carry on your body, the fat that threatens your very existence. If you want to live longer and more healthily, keeping that fat is simply not an option.

I hope that you will continue to eat the *Flat Belly Diet* way for as long as it takes for you to experience the freedom that comes from a healthier body weight. If you end up with abs of steel, I will be over-the-moon thrilled for you! (Although maybe just a teeny bit jealous.) But I'd be just as happy if you were to tell me that you finally lost your pregnancy weight, or you started walking or lowered your blood pressure, or you stopped buying shapeless, oversized tunics because you no longer feel self-conscious about the way you look. This plan is less about achieving an ideal body than it is about creating a healthier life. If you remember nothing about the *Flat Belly Diet* but the fact that a MUFA at every meal could save your life, then I've done my job. And you've done yours.

Conversion Charts

These equivalents have been slightly rounded to make measuring easier.

VOLUME MEASUREMENTS

U.S.	Imperial	Metric
¼tsp	–	1ml
½tsp	–	2ml
1tsp	–	5ml
1tbsp	–	15ml
2tbsp (1oz)	1floz	30ml
¼ cup (2oz)	2floz	60ml
1/3 cup (3oz)	3floz	80ml
½ cup (4oz)	4floz	120ml
2/3 cup (5oz)	5floz	160ml
¾ cup (6oz)	6floz	180ml
1 cup (8oz)	8floz	240ml

PAN SIZES

U.S.	Metric
8in cake pan	20 x 4cm sandwich or cake tin
9in cake pan	23 x 3.5cm sandwich or cake tin
11 x 7in baking pan	28 x 18cm baking tin
13 x 9in baking pan	32.5 x 23cm baking tin
15 x 10in baking pan	38 x 25.5cm baking tin (Swiss roll tin)
1½ quart baking dish	1.5 litre baking dish
2 quart baking dish	2 litre baking dish
2 quart rectangular baking dish	30 x 19cm baking dish
9in pie plate	22 x 4 or 23 x 4cm pie plate
7 or 8in springform pan	18 or 20cm springform or loose-bottom cake tin
9 x 5in loaf pan	23 x 13cm or 2lb narrow loaf tin or pâté tin

Weight Measurements

U.S.	Metric
1oz	30g
2oz	60g
4oz (¼lb)	115g
5oz (⅓lb)	145g
6oz	170g
7oz	200g
8oz (½lb)	230g
10oz	285g
12oz (¾lb)	340g
14oz	400g
16oz (1lb)	450g
2¼lb	1kg

Temperatures

Fahrenheit	Centigrade	Gas
140°	60°	–
160°	70°	–
180°	80°	–
225°	105°	¼
250°	120°	½
275°	135°	1
300°	150°	2
325°	160°	3
350°	180°	4
375°	190°	5
400°	200°	6
425°	220°	7
450°	230°	8
475°	245°	9
500°	260°	–

Length Measurements

U.S.	Metric
¼in	0.6cm
½in	1.25cm
1in	2.5cm
2in	5cm
4in	10cm
8in	20cm
10in	25cm
12in (1ft)	30cm

endnotes

Chapter 1

1. J.A. Paniagua, A. Gallego de la Sacristana, I. Romero, A. Vidal-Puig, J.M. Latre, E. Sanchez, P. Perez-Martinez, J. Lopez-Miranda and F. Perez-Jimenez, 'Monounsaturated Fat–Rich Diet Prevents Central Body Fat Distribution and Decreases Postprandial Adiponectin Expression Induced by a Carbohydrate-Rich Diet in Insulin-Resistant Subjects', *Diabetes Care*, 30 (2007):1717–23.

Chapter 2

1. R.E. Ostlund, M. Staten, W.M. Kohrt, J. Schultz and M. Malley, 'The Ratio of Waist-to-Hip Circumference, Plasma Insulin Level, and Glucose Intolerance as Independent Predictors of the HDL2 Cholesterol Level in Older Adults', *New England Journal of Medicine*, 322, no. 4 (January 25, 1990):229–34.
2. László B. Tankó, Yu Z. Bagger, Peter Alexandersen, Philip J. Larsen, Claus Christiansen, 'Peripheral Adiposity Exhibits an Independent Dominant Antiatherogenic Effect in Elderly Women', *Circulation*, 107 (2003):1626.
3. Frank B. Hu; Tricia Y. Li; Graham A. Colditz; Walter C. Willett; JoAnn E. Manson, 'Television Watching and Other Sedentary Behaviors in Relation to Risk of Obesity and Type 2 Diabetes Mellitus in Women', *JAMA*, 289 (2003):1785–91.
4. R.A. Whitmer, S. Sidney, J. Selby, S. Claiborne Johnston and K. Yaffe, 'Midlife Cardiovascular Risk Factors and Risk of Dementia in Late Life', *Neurology*, 64 (2005):277–81.
5. http://win.niddk.nih.gov/publications/tools.htm#circumf.
6. http://www.rush.edu/itools/hip/hipcalc.html.
7. 'Thin People May Be Obese on the Inside', *Medical Research News*, 14 May, 2007, reporting a study funded by the Medical Research Council under the direction of Dr Jimmy Bell, professor of molecular imaging at Imperial College, London, http://www.news-medical.net/?id=25076.
8. Salim Yusuf, Steven Hawken, et al. 'Obesity and the Risk of Myocardial Infarction in 27,000 Participants from 52 Countries; A Case-Control Study', *Lancet*, 366 (2005):1640–49.
9. 'Modest Gain in Visceral Fat Causes Dysfunction of Blood Vessel Lining in Lean Healthy Humans; Shedding Weight Restores Vessel

Health', presented by the Mayo Clinic team at the American Heart Association's Scientific Sessions, November 2007, http://www. sciencedaily.com/releases/2007/11/071105121934.htm.

Chapter 3

1. S. J. Nicholls, P. Lundman, J. A. Harmer, B. Cutri, K. A. Griffiths, K. A. Rye, P. J. Barter and D. S. Celermajer, 'Consumption of Saturated Fat Impairs the Anti-inflammatory Properties of High-Density Lipoproteins and Endothelial Function', *Journal of the American College of Cardiology*, 48, no. 4 (2006):715–20.

2. David Kritchevsky, 'History of Recommendations to the Public about Dietary Fat', *The Journal of Nutrition*, 128, no. 2 (1998):449S–452S.

3. National Advisory Committee on Nutrition Education. A Discussion Paper on Proposals for Nutritional Guidelines for Health Education in Britain. London: Health Education Council, 1983.

4. Department of Health. Nutritional Aspects of Cardiovascular Disease. Report of the Cardiovascular Review Group of the Committee on Medical Aspects of Food Policy. Report on Health and Social Subjects 46. London: HMSO, 1994.

5 DEFRA (2001) National Food Survey 2000. The Stationery Office. London.

6. A. Keys, C. Aravanis, H. W. Blackburn, F. S. Van Buchem, R. Buzina, B. D. Djordjevic, A. S. Dontas, F. Fidanza, M. J. Karvonen, N. Kimura, D. Lekos, M. Monti, V. Puddu, and H. L Taylor, 'Epidemiological Studies Related to Coronary Heart Disease: Characteristics of Men Aged 40–59 in Seven Countries', *Acta Medica Scandinavica Supplementum*, 460 (1966):1–392.

7. M. D. Kontogianni, D. B. Panagiotakos, C. Chrysohoou, C. Pitsavos, A. Zampelas and C. Stefanadis, 'The Impact of Olive Oil Consumption Pattern on the Risk of Actute Coronary Syndromes: The CARDIO2000 Case-Control Study', *Clinical Cardiology*, 30, no. 3 (2007):125–9.

8. H. M. Roche, A. Zampelas, J. M. Knapper, D. Webb, C. Brooks, K. G. Jackson, J. W. Wright, B. J. Gould, A. Kafatos, M. J. Gibney and C. M. Williams, 'Effect of Long-Term Olive Oil Dietary Intervention on Postprandial Triacylglycerol and Factor VII Metabolism', *American Journal of Clinical Nutrition*, 68, no. 3 (1998):552–60.

9. W. R. Archer, B. Lamarche, A. C. St-Pierre, J. F. Mauger, O. Deriaz, N. Landry, L. Corneau, J. P. Despres, J. Bergeron, J. Couture and N. Bergeron, 'High Carbohydrate and High Monounsaturated Fatty Acid Diets Similarly Affect LDL Electrophoretic Characteristics in Men Who Are Losing Weight', *Journal of Nutrition*, 133, no. 10 (2003):3124–9.

10. L. J. Appel, F. M. Sacks, V. J. Carey, E. Obarzanek, J. F. Swain, E. R. Miller III, P. R. Conlin, T. P. Erlinger, B. A. Rosner, N. M. Laranjo, J. Charleston, P. McCarron and L. M. Bishop, OmniHeart Collaborative Research Group, 'Effects of Protein, Monounsaturated Fat, and Carbohydrate Intake on Blood Pressure and Serum Lipids: Results of the Omniheart Randomized Trial', *The Journal of the American Medical Association*, 294, no. 19 (2005):2455–64.

11. P. M. Kris-Etherton, T. A. Pearson, Y. Wan, R. L. Hargrove, K. Moriarty, V. Fishell and T. D. Etherton, 'High-Monounsaturated Fatty Acid Diets Lower Both Plasma Cholesterol and Triacylglycerol Concentrations', *American Journal of Clinical Nutrition*, 70, no. 6 (1999):1009–15.

12. R. Estruch, M. A. Martinez-Gonzalez, D. Corella, J. Salas-Salvado, V. Ruiz-Gutierrez, M. I. Covas, M. Fiol, E. Gomez-Gracia, M. C. Lopez-Sabater, E. Vinyoles, F. Aros, M. Conde, C. Hahoz, J. Lapetra, G. Saez and E. Ros, PREDIMED Study Investigators, 'Effects of a Mediterranean-Style Diet on Cardiovascular Risk Factors: A Randomized Trial', *Annals of Internal Medicine*, 145, no. 1 (2006):1–11.

13. J. A. Paniagua, A. Gallego de la Sacristana, I. Romero, A. Vidal-Puig, J. M. Latre, E. Sanchez, P. Perez-Martinez, J. Lopez-Miranda and F. Perez-Jimenez, 'Monounsaturated Fat-Rich Diet Prevents Central Body Fat Distribution and Decreases Postprandial Adiponectin Expression Induced by a Carbohydrate-Rich Diet in Insulin-Resistant Subjects', *Diabetes Care*, 30, no. 7 (2007):1717–23.

14. B. Gumbiner, C. C. Low and P. D. Reaven, 'Effects of a Monounsaturated Fatty Acid-Enriched Hypocaloric Diet on Cardiovascular Risk Factors in Obese Patients with Type 2 Diabetes', *Diabetes Care*, 21, no. 1 (1998):9–15.

15. C. Romero, E. Medina, J. Vargas, M. Brenes and A. De Castro, 'In Vitro Activity of Olive Oil Polyphenols against *Helicobacter pylori*', *Journal of Agriculture and Food Chemistry*, 55, no. 3 (2007):680–686.

16. G. Zhao, T. D. Etherton, K. R. Martin, S. G. West, P. J. Gillies and P. M. Kris-Etherton, 'Dietary Alpha-Linolenic Acid Reduces Inflammatory and Lipid Cardiovascular Risk Factors in

Hypercholesterolemic Men and Women', *Journal of Nutrition,* 134 (2004):2991–2997.

17. N. Z. Unlu, T. Bohn, S. K. Clinton and S. J. Schwartz, 'Carotenoid Absorption from Salad and Salsa by Humans Is Enhanced by the Addition of Avocado or Avocado Oil', *The Journal of Nutrition,* 135, no. 3 (2005):431–436.

18. L. Berglund, M. Lefebre, H. N. Ginsberg, P. M. Kris-Etherton, P. J. Elmer, P. W. Stewart, A. Ershow, T. A. Pearson, B. H. Dennis, P. S. Roheim, R. Ramakrishnan, R. Reed, K. Stewart and K. M. Phillips, DELTA Investigators, 'Comparison of Monounsaturated Fat with Carbohydrates as a Replacement for Saturated Fat in Subjects with a High Metabolic Risk Profile: Studies in the Fasting and Postprandial States', *American Journal of Clinical Nutrition,* 86, no. 6 (2007): 611–20.

19. J. Salas-Salvado, A. Garcia-Arellano, F. Estruch, F. Marquez-Sandoval, D. Corella, M. Fiol, E. Gomez-Gracia, E. Vinoles, F. Aros, C. Herrera, C. Lahoz, J. Lapetra, J. S. Perona, D. Munoz-Aguado, M. A. Martinez-Gonzalez and E. Ros, 'Components of the Mediterranean-Type Food Pattern and Serum Inflammatory Markers among Patients at High Risk for Cardiovascular Disease', *European Journal of Clinical Nutrition,* advance online publication doi: 10.1038/sj.ejcn.1602762 (18 April 2007), www.nature.com/ejcn/journal/vaop/ncurrent/abs/1602762a.html.

20. K. Esposito, R. Marfella, M. Ciotola, C. Di Palo, F. Giugliano, G. Fiugliano, M. D'Armiento, F. D'Andrea and D. Giugliano, 'Effect of a Mediterranean-Style Diet on Endothelial Dysfunction and Markers of Vascular Inflammation in the Metabolic Syndrome: A Randomized Trial', *The Journal of the American Medical Association,* 292, no. 12 (2004):1440–6.

21. A. Wolk, R. Bergstrom, D. Hunter, W. Willett, H. Ljung, L. Holmberg, L. Bergkvist, A. Bruce and H. O. Adami, 'A Prospective Study of Association of Monounsaturated Fat and Other Types of Fat with Risk of Breast Cancer', *Archives of Internal Medicine,* 158, no. 1 (1998):41–5.

22. V. Solfrizzi, F. Panza, F. Torres, F. Mastroianni, A. Del Parigi, A. Venezia and A. Capurso, 'High Monounsaturated Fatty Acids Intake Protects against Age-Related Cognitive Decline', *Neurology,* 52, no. 8 (1999):1563–9.

23. F. Panza, V. Solfrizzi, A. M. Colacicco, A. D'Introno, C. Capurso, F.

Torres, A. Del Parigi, S. Capurso and A. Capurso, 'Mediterranean Diet and Cognitive Decline', *Public Health Nutrition*, 7, no. 7 (2004):959–63.

24. V. Solfrizzi, A. D'Introno, A. M. Colacicco, C. Capurso, R. Palasciano, S. Capurso, F. Torres, A. Capurso and F. Panza, 'Unsaturated Fatty Acids Intake and All-Causes Mortality: A 8.5-Year Follow-Up of the Italian Longitudinal Study on Aging', *Experimental Gerontology*, 40, no. 4 (2005):335–43.

25. J. A. Paniagua, A. Gallego dl la Sacristana, I. Romero, A. Vidal-Puig, J. M. Latre, E. Sanchez, P. Perez-Martinez, J. Lopez-Miranda, F. Perez-Jimenez, 'Monounsaturated Fat-Rich Diet Prevents Central Body Fat Distribution and Decreases Postprandial Adiponectin Expression Induced by a Carbohydrate-Rich Diet in Insulin-Resistant Subjects', *Diabetes Care*, 3, no. 7 (2007):1717–23.

26. L. S. Piers, K. Z. Walker, R. M. Stoney, M. J. Soares and K. O'Dea, 'The Influence of the Type of Dietary Fat on Postprandial Fat Oxidation Rates: Monounsaturated (Olive Oil) vs. Saturated Fat (Cream)', *International Journal of Obesity and Related Metabolic Disorders*, 26, no. 6 (2002):814–21.

Chapter 4

1. Doreen Virtue, *Constant Craving A–Z* (Carlsbad, CA: Hay House, 1999).

2. Jennifer A. Linde, Robert W. Jeffery, Simone A. French, Nicolaas P. Pronk, Raymond G. Boyle, 'Self-Weighing in Weight Gain Prevention and Weight Loss Trials', *Annals of Behavioral Medicine*, 30, no. 3 (2005):210–16.

3. http://www.foodandmood.org/Pages/sh-survey.html

4. Mikko Laaksonen, Sirpa Sarlio-Lähteenkorva, Päivi Leino-Arjas, Pekka Martikainen and Eero Lahelma, 'Body Weight and Health Status: Importance of Socioeconomic Position and Working Conditions', *Obesity Research*, 13 (2005):2169–77.

5. Jos A. Bosch, Eco J.C. de Geus, Angele Kelder, Enno C.I. Veerman, Johan Hoogstraten and Arie V. Nieuw Amerongen, 'Differential Effects of Active versus Passive Coping on Secretory Immunity', *Psychophysiology*, 38, no. 5 (2001), doi:10.1111/1469–8986.3850836.

6. Ann Hettinger, 'Rest Assured', *Prevention*, 59, no. 12 (December 2007):48.

7. Ann Hettinger, 'Rest Assured', *Prevention*, 59, no. 12 (December 2007):48.

8. D. L. Sherrill, K. Kotchou, S. F. Quan, 'Association of Physical Activity and Human Sleep Disorders', *Archives of Internal Medicine*, 158, no. 17 (28 September, 1998):1894–98, http://archinte.ama-assn.org/cgi/reprint/158/17/1894.

Chapter 5

1. Philip S. Chua, 'Air Travel: Medical Tips', *Heart to Heart Talk, CEBU Cardiovascular Center* (2003), http://www.cebudoctorsuniversity.edu/hospital/cardio/chua2.html.

2. J. W. Pennebaker, J. K. Kiecolt-Glaser and R. Glaser, 'Disclosure of Traumas and Immune Function: Health Implications for Psychotherapy', *Journal of Consulting and Clinical Psychology*, 56 (1988):239–45.

Chapter 7

1. Steven Reinberg, 'Excess Pounds Raise Women's Cancer Risk', *HealthDay* (November 7, 2007), http://body.aol.com/condition-center/breast-cancer/news/article/_a/excess-pounds-raise-womens-cancer-risk/n20071107090309990041.

Chapter 9

1. I. Giannopoulou, L. L. Ploutz-Snyder, R. Carhart, R. S. Weinstock, B. Fernhall, S. Goulopoulou and J. A. Kanaley, 'Exercise Is Required for Visceral Fat Loss in Postmenopausal Women with Type 2 Diabetes', *Journal of Clinical Endocrinology & Metabolism*, 90, no. 3 (2005):1511–18.

2. S. K. Park, J. H. Park, Y. C. Kwon, H. S. Kim, M. S. Yoon and H. T. Park, 'The Effect of Combined Aerobic and Resistance Exercise Training on Abdominal Fat in Obese Middle-Aged Women', *Journal of Physiological Anthropology and Applied Human Science*, 22, no. 3 (May 2003):129–35.

3. Melinda L. Irwin, Yutaka Yasui, Cornelia M. Ulrich, Deborah Bowen, Rebecca E. Rudolph, Robert S. Schwartz, Michi Yukawa, Erin Aiello,

John D. Potter and Anne McTiernan, 'Effect of Exercise on Total and Intra-abdominal Body Fat in Postmenopausal Women', *JAMA*, 289 (2003):323–30.

4. 'Depression and Anxiety: Exercise Eases Symptoms', *MayoClinic.com* (October 23, 2006), http://www.mayoclinic.com/health/depression-and-exercise/MH00043.

5. Anne J. Blood and Robert J. Zatorre, 'Intensely Pleasurable Responses to Music Correlate with Activity in Brain Regions Implicated in Reward and Emotion', *Proceedings of the National Academy of Sciences*, 98, no. 20 (25 September, 2001):11818–23.

6. Charles F. Emery, Evana T. Hsiao, Scott M. Hill and David J. Frid, 'Short-Term Effects of Exercise and Music on Cognitive Performance among Participants in a Cardiac Rehabilitation Program', *Heart & Lung: The Journal of Acute and Critical Care*, 32, issue 6 (November/December 2003):368–73.

Chapter 10

1. 'With Obesity on the Rise, Dieting a Constant Concern', *Calorie Control*, 29 (Autumn 2007), http://www.caloriecontrol.org/pdf/ccc%20comm%20fall07_3.pdf.

2. Willard Bishop, 'Making Healthy Eating Easier', *Shopping for Health 2006*, survey by *Prevention* magazine (2006).

3. M. L. Irwin, Y. Yasui, C. M. Ulrich, D. Bowen, R. E. Rudolph, R. S. Schwartz, M. Yukawa, E. Aiello, J. D. Potter, A. McTiernan, 'Effect of Exercise on Total and Intra-abdominal Body Fat in Postmenopausal Women: A Randomized Controlled Trial', *JAMA*, 289, no. 3 (15 January, 2003):323–30, http://jama.ama-assn.org/cgi/content/full/289/3/323?ijkey=2ffd96d981677fb09007213e18cda542e6ed4cc0.

index

Headings in *italic* indicate recipes and easy meals. Page numbers in **bold** indicate text in shaded or other boxes, and those followed by 'Q' show question sections.